耳鼻咽喉科学聚焦

ENT in Focus

IN*focus*

注　意

医学知识总是在不断进展。疾病的诊治应当遵循一定的成规，然而随着新的研究和临床经验不断扩大我们的知识面，合理地改变治疗方法与临床用药也是必要的。读者在实际用药过程中，应当先查看药物生产厂家所提供的说明书，以便掌握药物的推荐剂量、用药途径、服药周期以及药物的禁忌证。临床医师有责任根据既往经验以及患者的实际情况来为每一位患者制定出最适宜的治疗方案和用药剂量。本书出版方及作者均不对本读物引起的人员损伤或财产损失负责。

出版者

耳鼻咽喉科学聚焦

ENT in Focus

IN*focus*

原　著　Robin Youngs

Nicholas D Stafford

主　译　肖水芳　邓　达

译　者　（以姓氏笔画为序）

王全桂　邓　达　陈　剑

肖水芳　钟　贞

秘　书　杨　柳

北京大学医学出版社

Peking University Medical Press

北京市版权局著作权合同登记号：图字：**01-2006-1814**

原著书名 **ENT in Focus**
原作者 **Robin Youngs, Nicholas D Stafford**
ISBN-13: **978-0-443-10080-2**
ISBN-10: **0-443-10080-2**

978-981-259-557-7
981-259-557-0

Elsevier (Singapore) Pte Ltd.
3 Killiney Road, #08-01 Winsland House I, Singapore 239519
Tel: (65) 6349-0200, Fax: (65) 6733-1817
First Published **2009**
2009 年初版

图书在版编目（CIP）数据

耳鼻咽喉科学聚焦 /（英）扬斯（Youngs，R.），（英）斯塔福德（Stafford，N. D.）原著；肖水芳，邓达译. —北京：北京大学医学出版社，2009

书名原文：ENT in Focus

ISBN 978-7-81116-282-0

Ⅰ. 耳…　Ⅱ. ①扬… ②斯… ③肖… ④邓…　Ⅲ. 耳鼻咽喉病—诊疗　Ⅳ. R76

中国版本图书馆 CIP 数据核字（2008）第 145385 号

耳鼻咽喉科学聚焦

主　　译：肖水芳　邓　达

出版发行：北京大学医学出版社 (电话：010-82802230)

地　　址：(100191) 北京市海淀区学院路 38 号　北京大学医学部院内

网　　址：http://www.pumpress.com.cn

E-mail：booksale@bjmu.edu.cn

印　　刷：莱芜市圣龙印务有限责任公司

经　　销：新华书店

责任编辑：陈　碧　　**责任校对**：杜　悦　　**责任印制**：郭桂兰

开　　本：889mm × 1194mm　1/32　　**印张**：9　　**字数**：229 千字

版　　次：2009 年 1 月第 1 版　2009 年 1 月第 1 次印刷

书　　号：ISBN 978-7-81116-282-0

定　　价：68.00 元

译者前言

耳鼻咽喉头颈外科学不同于其他学科的特点之一是其器官多位于头面和颈部的骨性、软骨性或肌性的管道或腔隙中，常需要借助相应的检查方法和特殊器械方可窥及。这对于医学生、社区医师和低年住院医师是一个不小的挑战。Youngs博士和Stafford教授主编的《耳鼻咽喉科学聚焦》用简明的语言辅以精美高清晰图片对耳鼻咽喉头颈外科常见的疾病从病原学、发病原理、临床特征和治疗进行了图文并茂的阐述。

该书的第一部分涵盖了该学科临床医学教育的基本内容，其中众多精美临床照片是对传统医学教科书的一个很好的补充。在内容编排上，突出以临床病例为主线，大致按照耳、鼻、咽、喉、头颈和口腔疾病的顺序编写了50章节的精彩内容，读者可在较短时间内浏览众多病例，其中很多病例在医学生有限的实习期内是不可能看到的。该书的第二部分内容是以临床解剖标本，临床病例所见，鼻内镜、耳内镜或纤维内镜下所见，X线、CT等影像学资料以及听力学的一些基本检查方法为主线，编辑了71个自测题。每道题有1至4个小问题，每个问题都配有1张或2张清晰图片或照片，共74张。这些问题是为了让读者自测对第一部分内容的学习掌握情况，可为临床考试做准备。该书的最后一部分内容是自测题的参考答案。借此，读者可自我评估对所学知识的掌握程度。三部分内容前呼后应，构成了一套完整的自学自测教材。

该书1988年第一次以《ENT彩色助手》的书名出版，1994年改为《ENT彩色指南》再版，1999年《ENT彩色指南》第二版出版，2005年第一次以《ENT聚焦》作为临床医学教育十个二级学科系列出版物之一出版发行。目前国内教科书中尚缺少专门面向医学生、社区医师和低年住院医师的同类出版物，相信该书中文译本的出版发行对上述读者群体的临床医学学习将有所裨益。

该书在选题和编辑过程中得到北京大学医学出版社王凤廷副社长、陈碧编辑的悉心指导和协助，借此表达我们的敬意和谢意。

鉴于译者的水平，翻译过程中的偏差之处，恳请读者和同道们海涵并指正。

肖水芳
中华医学会耳鼻咽喉头颈科学分会常务委员
北京大学第一临床医院耳鼻咽喉头颈外科主任
2008-9-18

致　谢

作者向以下为本书提供素材的单位表示感谢：伦敦圣玛丽医院医学影像科、伦敦St Bartholomew医院图片资料科以及Ipswich医院。同时向Wright先生（图52、64及87）、Choy医师（图35、41）、Lissauer医师（图106、140及156）、Archer先生（图95及165）、Breach先生（图13）、Davies先生（图160）、Eyre先生（图116）、Forge医师（图54）、Henk医师（图120）及Rhys-Evans先生（图121）等表示感谢。作者特别感谢Michael Hawke教授所提供的优质显微耳镜照片（图9、15、17、23、27及34）。最后，向本书照片中所涉及到的所有患者致谢！没有他们的配合，本书将无法顺利完成。

目录

Contents

耳镜检查

用耳镜检查耳部时也应该观察外耳的各种异常情况，包括既往中耳手术所遗留的瘢痕。外耳道呈S型，检查外耳道时将耳廓向后上牵拉以使其变直，这样做在大多数情况下可以很好地观察到鼓膜（图1）。正常的鼓膜呈灰白色、半透明，可以看见位居中央部位的锤骨柄（图2）。下部的鼓膜非常薄，我们称之为鼓膜的紧张部。上部的皮肤较厚，我们称之为鼓膜的松弛部。

音叉试验

可以用一个512Hz的音叉来粗略地评估听力（图3）。用Rinne和Weber试验可以区别是由中耳疾病引起的传导性聋，还是由内耳疾病引起的感音神经性聋。

听力计检查

纯音测听用来检查不同频率纯音的听阈（图4）。声阻抗检查用以测量耳道不同压力下鼓膜的顺应性。用这种方法可以评估中耳的压力并判断出中耳积液的存在。

Assessment of the ear

Otoscopy

The external ear should be inspected for abnormalities, which may include scars from previous middle ear surgery. The external ear canal is S-shaped and can be straightened by upward and backward traction on the pinna, giving a good view of the tympanic membrane in most cases (Fig. 1). The normal tympanic membrane has a grey, translucent appearance with the handle of the malleus visible centrally (Fig. 2). The lower part of the membrane is very thin and is known as the pars tensa. In the upper part the skin is thicker and is known as the pars flaccida.

Tuning fork tests

A 512Hz tuning fork can be used to crudely assess hearing (Fig. 3). Using the Rinne and Weber tests, a diagnosis of conductive deafness due to middle ear disease can be distinguished from sensorineural deafness due to inner ear disease.

Audiometry

Pure tone audiometry is used to measure the threshold of hearing across a range of frequencies (Fig. 4). Impedance audiometry measures the compliance of the tympanic membrane in response to changing pressure in the ear canal. In this way middle ear pressure and the presence of middle ear fluid can be assessed.

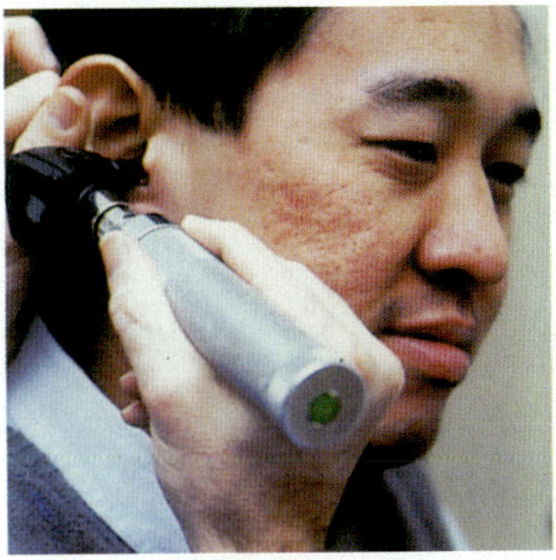

图 1　用耳镜检查耳部
Examination of the ear with an otoscope.

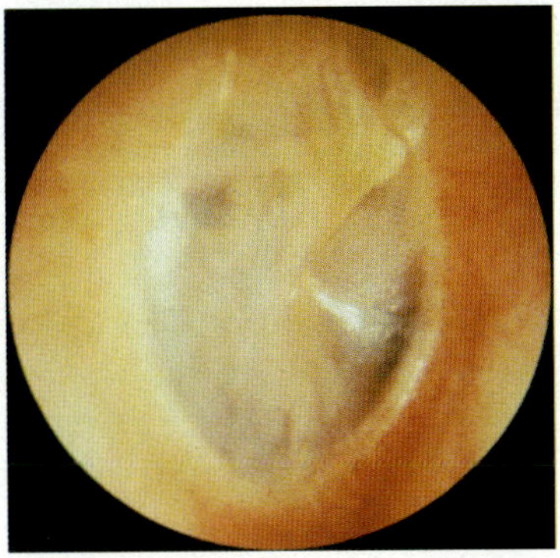

图 2　正常鼓膜
Normal tympanic membrane.

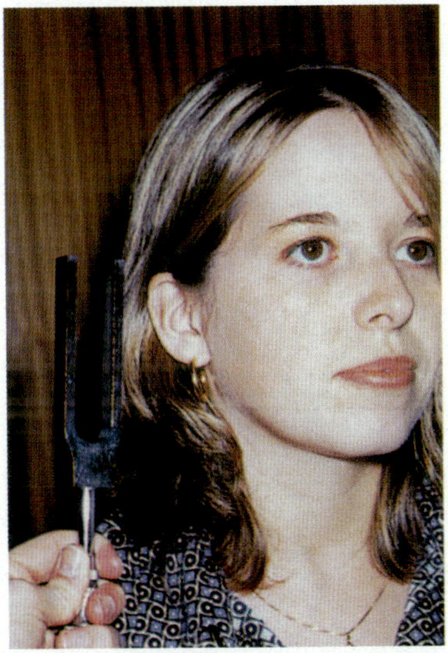

图 3　Rinne 音叉试验检查听力
Rinne's tuning fork test of hearing.

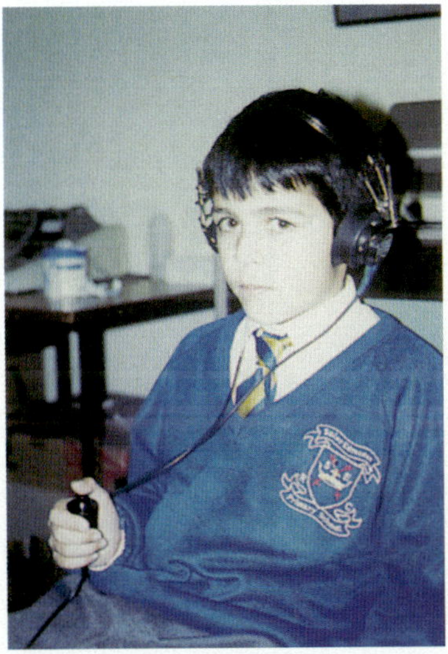

图 4　纯音测听
Pure tone audiometry.

2 耳的先天性疾病

外耳

临床特征

耳廓可能缺失或发育不全（小耳畸形）(图5)，第一鳃裂闭合不全将导致先天性耳前瘘管，其瘘口常见于耳轮脚前或耳屏前（图6)。耳前瘘管若发生感染则需切除。副耳可能出现在正常耳廓附近（图7)。

中耳

临床特征

听骨链的缺失常常与外耳道闭锁一同出现。Treacher-Collins综合征包括外、中耳畸形以及面骨发育异常。

治疗

骨锚式助听器（Bone Anchored Hearing Aids，BAHA）和耳廓假体（图8）的应用显著促进了对这类疾病的治疗，尤其是双侧病变的患者。BAHA即通过一个穿经皮肤的螺钉将助听器直接固定在颅骨上。

内耳

先天性的内耳缺陷往往导致严重的感音神经性聋。这类疾病可能有遗传基础。内耳的损害也可因孕期或围生期的损害造成，包括感染（尤其是母亲患风疹或梅毒)、新生儿溶血病以及分娩时胎儿缺氧。

治疗

先天性耳部疾患的治疗关键在于尽早地发现耳聋，这样就可以及时地给予治疗，使得患儿在儿童早期拥有良好的语言发育。

Congenital ear disease

External ear

Clinical features

The pinna may be absent or rudimentary (microtia) (Fig. 5). Failure of obliteration of the first branchial cleft results in a congenital sinus usually found in front of the helix or tragus (Fig. 6), which may become a site of infection requiring its excision. Accessory auricles can occur adjacent to a normally placed pinna (Fig. 7).

Middle ear

Clinical features

Ossicular chain defects often occur in association with atresia of the external auditory canal. Treacher-Collins syndrome consists of middle and external ear malformation with abnormal facial bone development.

Management

Bone anchored hearing aids and auricular prostheses (Fig. 8) have greatly improved the treatment of these conditions. particularly in bilateral cases. With this technique prostheses are secured directly to the bones of the skull via osseo-integrated screws passing through the skin.

Inner ear

Congenital defects of the inner ear usually result in severe sensorineural deafness. These disorders may have a hereditary basis. Damage to the inner ear can also be caused by events during pregnancy and the perinatal period. These include infections, particularly maternal rubella and syphilis, haemolytic disease of the newborn and fetal anoxia during birth.

Management

In the management of congenital ear disease it is vital that deafness, if present, is detected at an early stage so that treatment is instituted, allowing optimum language development during early childhood.

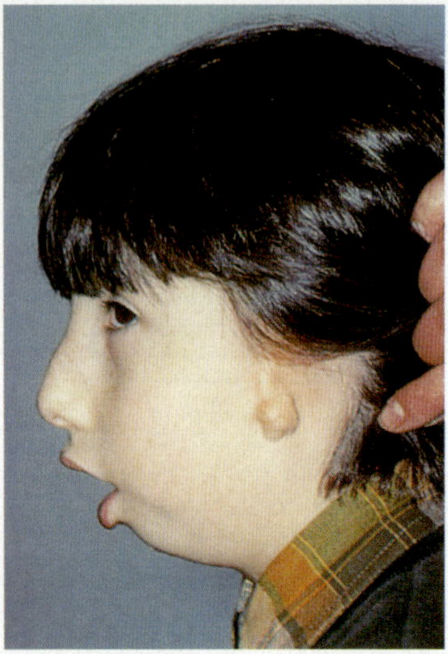

图 5　小耳畸形
Microtia.

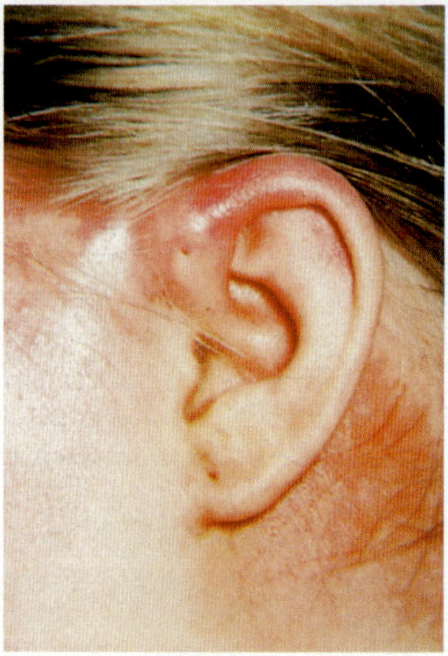

图 6　耳前瘘管
Preauricular sinus.

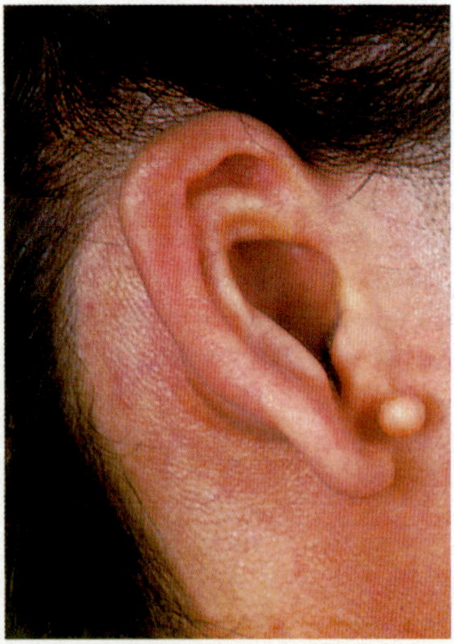

图 7　副耳
Accessory auricles.

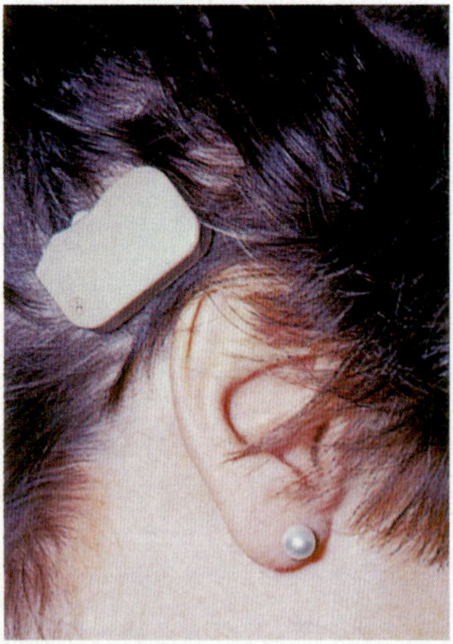

图 8　骨锚式助听器
Bone anchored hearing aid in place.

异物

临床特征 外耳异物最常见于儿童，异物可能是小珠子、棉绒团等(图 9)。如果异物插进外耳道过深，可能造成鼓膜穿孔(图 10)。

治疗 取出外耳道异物可能需要全麻。大多数外伤性鼓膜穿孔可以自行愈合。

菜花状耳

临床特征 耳廓的钝性创伤可以造成软骨膜下血肿（图 11)。由于缺乏血供，耳廓软骨出现坏死并被纤维组织所替代，从而形成菜花样的外耳畸形（图 12)。

治疗 早期对软骨膜下血肿进行引流通常可以避免畸形的发生。

软骨膜炎

开放性外伤或手术损伤累及耳廓软骨或外耳道软骨可能引起软骨膜炎。软骨膜炎有时也并发严重的外耳炎。

临床特征 临床表现为耳廓弥漫性的充血、疼痛和肿胀。肿胀可以造成外耳道狭窄。软骨膜炎还可以发展至严重的面部蜂窝织炎和软骨坏死。

治疗 应用抗生素，对脓肿进行外科引流。

3 External ear trauma

Foreign bodies

Clinical features

Foreign bodies are most commonly found in children, e.g. beads, cotton wool buds (Fig. 9). If deeply inserted into the external ear canal, they may cause tympanic membrane perforation (Fig. 10).

Management

Removal of foreign bodies may require a general anaesthetic. Most traumatic tympanic membrane perforations heal spontaneously.

Cauliflower ear

Clinical features

Blunt trauma to the pinna may produce a subperichondrial haematoma (Fig. 11). Devoid of its blood supply, the cartilage necroses and is replaced by fibrous tissue, resulting in an ugly cosmetic deformity (Fig. 12).

Management

Early drainage of the haematoma usually prevents any deformity.

Perichondritis

Perichondritis may result from open trauma, which may be surgical, involving the cartilage of the pinna or auditory meatus. Occasionally it complicates a severe otitis externa.

Clinical features

Presents as a generalized red, painful and tender swelling of the pinna and oedema may also stenose the meatus. A severe facial cellulitis and necrosis of the cartilage may develop.

Management

Treatment is with antibiotics and surgical drainage of any abscess.

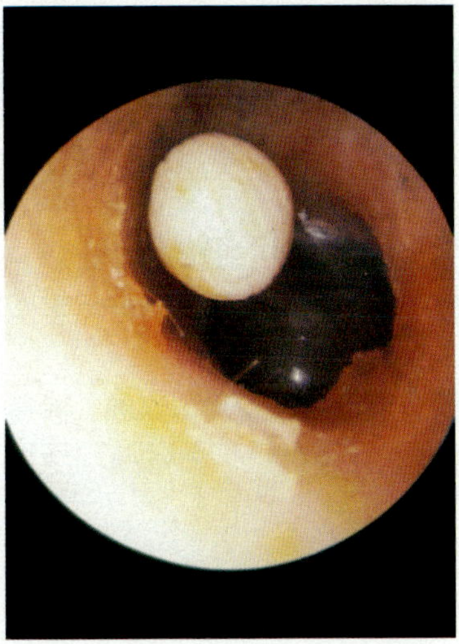

图 9　外耳道异物
Foreign body in the external canal.

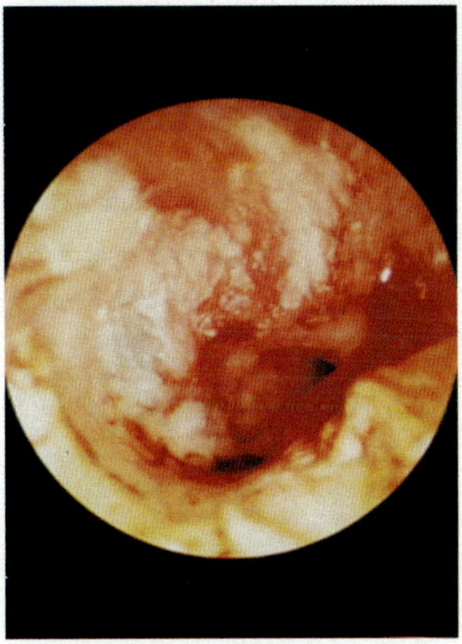

图 10　外伤性鼓膜穿孔
Traumatic perforation.

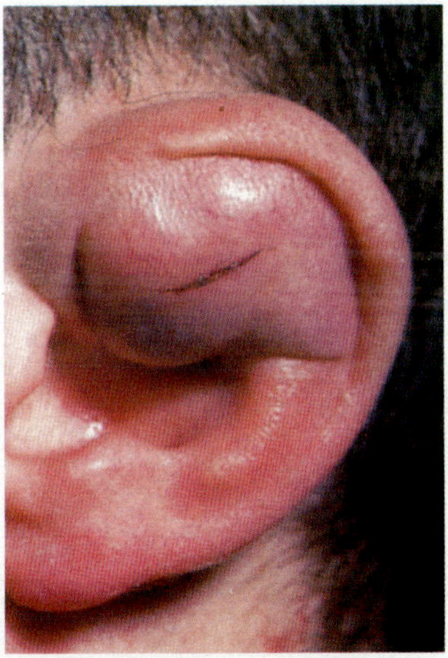

图 11　外伤后软骨膜下血肿
Subperichondrial haematoma due to trauma.

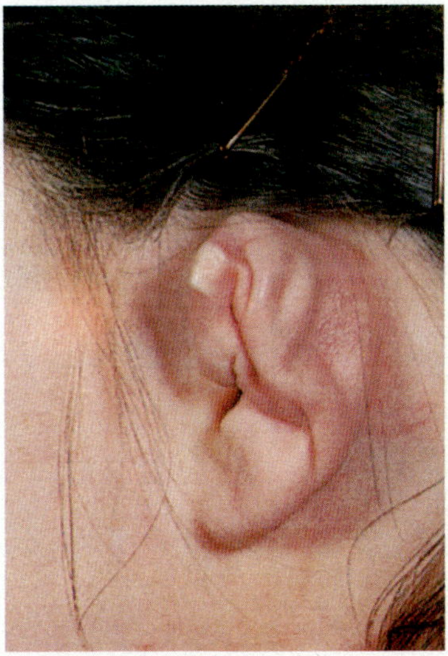

图 12　菜花状耳
Cauliflower ear.

恶性肿瘤

耳廓的皮肤可发生基底细胞癌、鳞状细胞癌（图 13）和恶性黑色素瘤。长时间暴露于阳光下是一个主要的危险因素。

临床特征 肿瘤最初呈小的、浅表的病变，后期发展呈深的、溃疡型病变。鳞癌和恶性黑色素瘤可以转移至区域颈淋巴结。

治疗 治疗方法为手术切除。基底细胞癌和鳞癌也可以用放疗。但侵及软骨的肿瘤对放射线敏感度降低。

良性肿瘤

外耳道骨性隆起是最常见的。

病因 骨瘤是单发的、真正的良性肿瘤。外生性骨疣通常是多发的，与游泳或跳水时外耳道反复暴露于冷水中有关。

临床特征 表现为骨部外耳道壁上光滑的隆起（图 14）。经常不引起任何临床症状，但如果外耳道腔被堵塞，则可能造成耵聍栓塞、外耳道炎或听力丧失。

治疗 如果没有症状则无需治疗。如果引起反复的外耳道炎，则需手术去除骨瘤。

Tumours of the pinna and external auditory meatus

4

Malignant tumours

Basal cell carcinomas, squamous cell carcinomas (Fig. 13) and malignant melanomas occur on the skin of the pinna. Exposure to sunlight over a long period is a major risk factor.

Clinical features

Initially small superficial lesions progressing to deep ulceration in advanced cases. Squamous carcinomas and malignant melanomas metastasize to regional cervical lymph nodes.

Management

Treated by surgical excision, although radiotherapy is an alternative for basal and squamous carcinomas. Involvement of cartilage renders the tumour less radiosensitive.

Benign tumours

Bony swellings of the external auditory meatus are most common.

Aetiology

Osteomas are solitary and are true benign neoplasms. Exostoses are usually multiple, being associated with repeated exposure of the external auditory canal to cold water as in swimming or diving.

Clinical features

Present as smooth swellings on the wall of the bony meatus (Fig.14). They are often asymptomatic but, if the lumen of the meatus is occluded, retention of wax, otitis externa or hearing loss may occur.

Management

None if asymptomatic. If recurrent otitis externa occurs, osteomas may be surgically reduced.

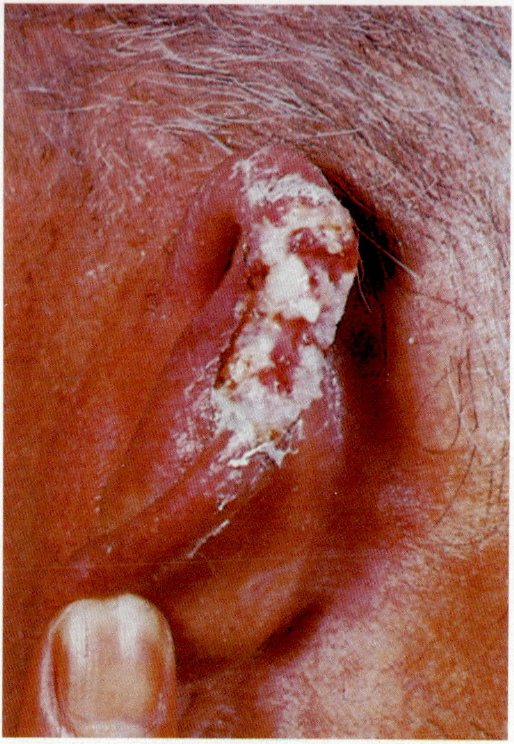

图 13　耳廓鳞癌
Squamous carcinoma of the pinna.

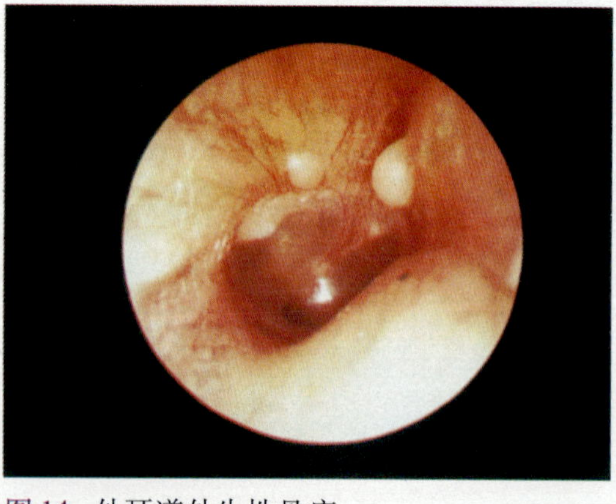

图 14　外耳道外生性骨疣
Exostoses of the external auditory canal.

外耳道炎

定义 外耳道皮肤的炎症。

病因 可以是原发的感染，也可是因外耳道皮肤局部接触化妆品或抗生素后过敏而引起的炎症。致病微生物常为革兰阴性菌（如变形杆菌、假单胞菌）和真菌（如曲霉）。引起该病的病因包括耵聍栓塞、局部损伤、中耳流脓经鼓膜穿孔引流至外耳道、游泳和一些皮肤病（如银屑病和脂溢性皮炎）。

临床特征 表现为耳痛、耳漏和耳聋。检查可见外耳道皮肤发炎、肿胀（图 15、16）。外耳道可被分泌物堵塞。如果是真菌感染，外耳道内可见菌丝（图 17）。牵拉耳廓可引起耳痛加重，这在中耳的感染中是不会出现的。

治疗 可以用干卷棉子擦拭或在手术显微镜下用吸引器清除外耳道内的碎屑和分泌物。在耳内滴用含抗生素和激素的滴耳液之前，应该用拭子取耳道内分泌物做细菌学检查。如果外耳道已经完全堵塞，可以将浸湿的小棉纱条插入外耳道。对于蜂窝织炎已经波及耳廓（图18）的严重病例，应全身应用抗生素治疗。

5 Otitis externa

Definition

Inflammation of the skin of the external auditory meatus.

Aetiology

Caused by either primary infection or contact sensitivity to topically applied substances such as cosmetics or antibiotics. Gram-negative organisms (e.g. *Proteus*, *Pseudomonas*) and fungi (e.g. *Aspergillus*) are often found. Precipitating factors include impacted cerumen, local trauma, middle ear discharge through a tympanic membrane perforation, swimming and skin conditions such as psoriasis and seborrhoeic dermatitis.

Clinical features

Presents as otalgia, otorrhoea and deafness. The skin of the external auditory meatus is oedematous and inflamed (Figs 15 & 16). The meatus may be occluded with discharge and in fungal infections hypae may be seen (Fig. 17). Traction on the pinna increases the otalgia, a sign not found in inflammatory conditions of the middle ear.

Management

Debris must be removed from the meatus, either by dry mopping or by suction aided by the use of an operating microscope. A swab of the meatus is taken for bacteriology prior to the instillation of drops containing an antibiotic and steroid mixture. If the meatus is totally occluded, an impregnated gauze wick may be inserted. In severe cases with cellulitis spreading onto the pinna (Fig. 18) systemic antibiotics are also needed.

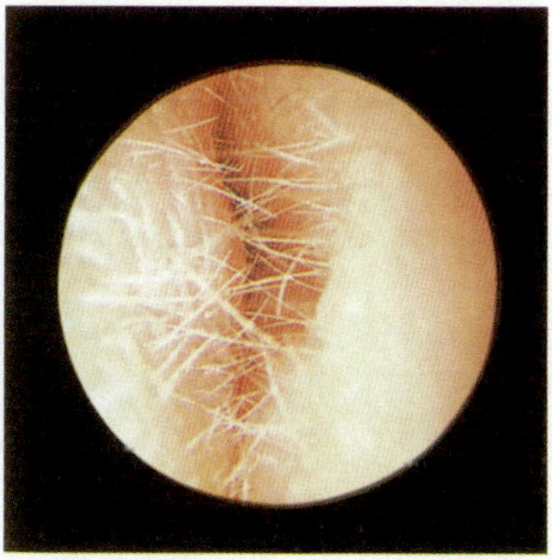

图 15 外耳炎合并耳道壁肿胀
Otitis externa with canal wall oedema.

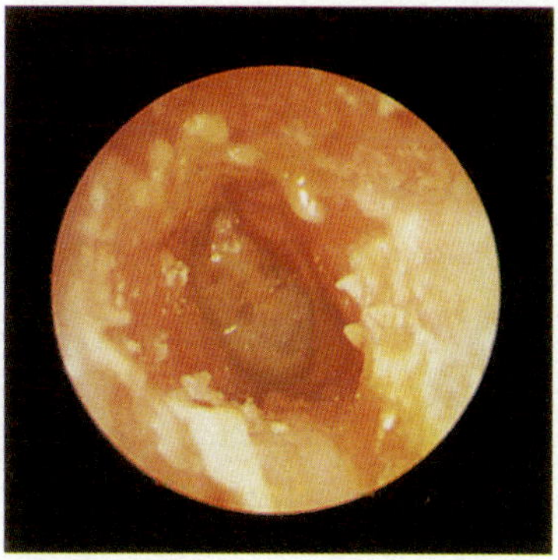

图 16 细菌性外耳炎
Bacterial otitis externa.

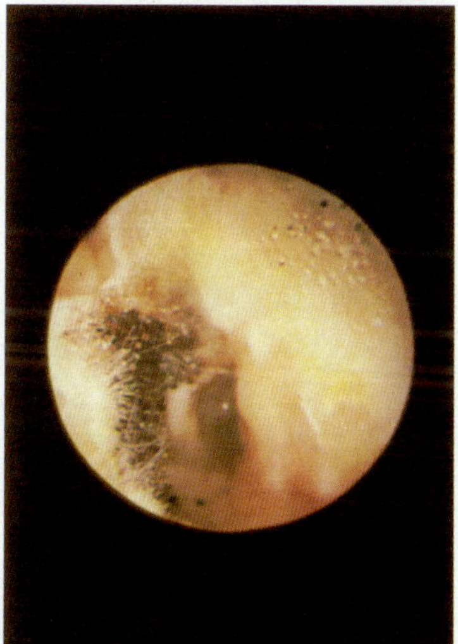

图 17 真菌性外耳炎
Fungal otitis externa.

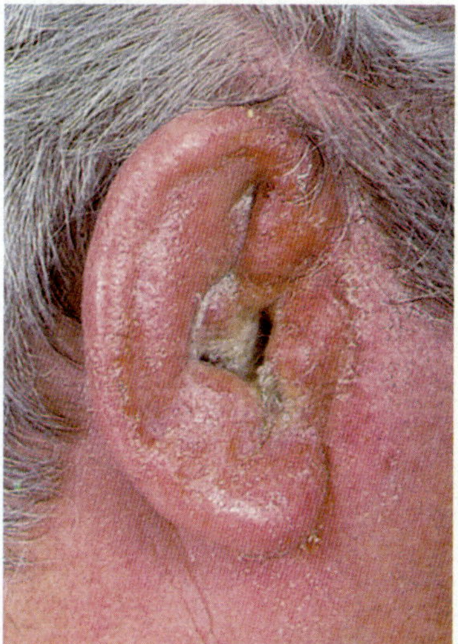

图 18 继发于外耳炎的耳廓蜂窝织炎
Cellulitis of the pinna secondary to otitis externa.

外耳道疖

外耳道软骨部毛囊的感染，常见病原为葡萄球菌。

临床特征 表现为严重的耳痛，牵拉耳廓时加重。如果耳道被疖肿堵塞可以出现耳聋。检查时可见外耳道内的疖肿。

治疗 多数疖肿可以自行破溃。可以将浸有甘油或鱼石脂的纱条塞入外耳道内进行治疗，每日更换一次（图 19）。全身可应用氟氯西林和止痛剂。

坏死性（恶性）外耳炎

是潜在致死性的外耳道假单胞菌感染，可以累及颅底。该病见于老年糖尿病患者，也可见于艾滋病患者。

临床特征 表现为严重的耳痛、耳漏和耳聋，严重的病例可导致脑神经（Ⅶ、Ⅸ、Ⅹ、Ⅺ、Ⅻ）麻痹。

治疗 治疗为局部手术治疗（通常是乳突切除术）联合超长疗程的特异性抗假单胞菌抗生素治疗。颅底的侵犯及治疗的疗效可以用同位素扫描的方法来评估（图 20）。

Furunculosis of the external auditory meatus

Staphylococcal infection of hair follicles found in the lateral part of the meatus.

Clinical features Presents as severe otalgia exacerbated by traction on the pinna, with deafness if the meatus becomes occluded. The furuncle is often visible.

Management Most furuncles rupture spontaneously. Ribbon gauze impregnated with glycerin/ichthammol may be inserted daily into the meatus (Fig. 19). Systemic flucloxacillin and analgesics are also needed.

Necrotizing (malignant) otitis externa

A potentially fatal Pseudomonas infection of the external auditory meatus, with spread to the skull base. It occurs in elderly diabetics and also in patients with HIV/AIDS.

Clinical features Presents as severe otalgia, otorrhoea and deafness with progression to cranial nerve palsies (VII, IX, X, XI, XII) in advanced cases.

Management Treatment is by local surgery, usually mastoidectomy, combined with a prolonged course of specific anti-pseudomonal antibiotics. Skull base involvement and its response to treatment may be assessed by radioisotope scanning (Fig. 20).

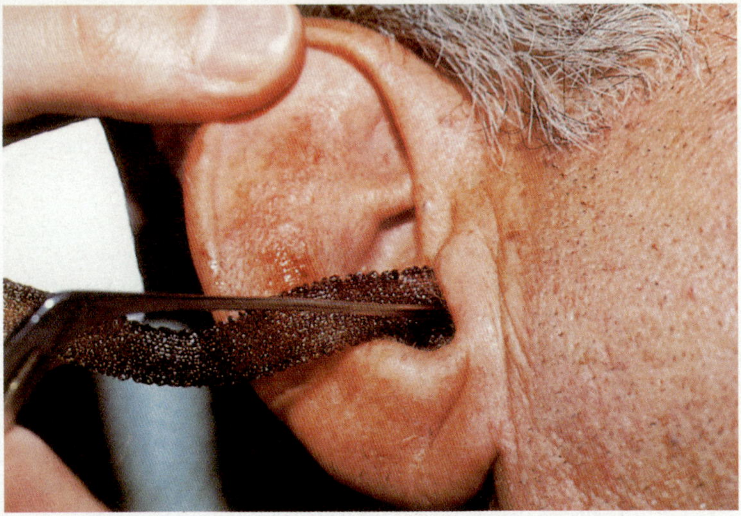

图 19 耳道内塞入浸有甘油和鱼石脂的纱条
Glycerin and ichthammol wick insertion.

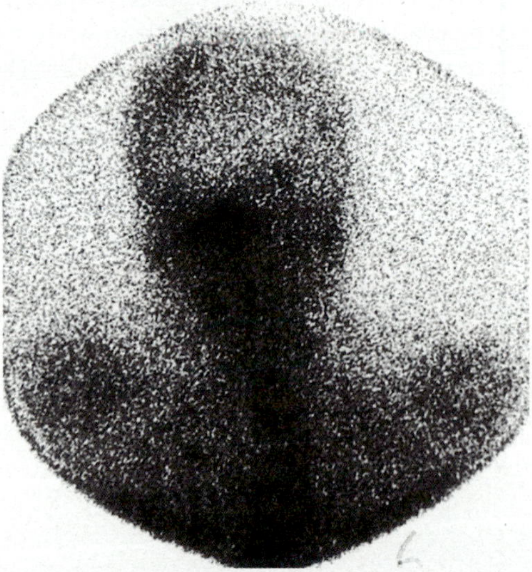

图 20 坏死性外耳道炎镓扫描：岩尖部可见同位素聚集增加
Gallium scan in necrotizing otitis externa: increased uptake at petrous apex.

大疱性鼓膜炎

病因

大疱性鼓膜炎由鼓膜和外耳道深部的流感病毒感染所致，常伴发急性中耳炎。

临床特征

表现为耳痛，听力下降和血清性耳溢液。耳镜检查可见鼓膜表面血疱（图 21）。若继发细菌感染可出现耳脓性溢液，也可导致外耳道炎。

治疗

用镇痛药治疗；若继发细菌感染，用局部或全身抗生素治疗。

鼓室硬化

病因

中耳炎或中耳手术，特别是鼓膜置管术后，鼓膜和中耳的黏膜下胶原沉淀而形成。

临床特征

鼓室硬化常无任何症状。胶原沉淀物表现为鼓膜表面白色的“粉笔灰”样的物质（图 22）。中耳的沉淀物可以引起听骨链固定而导致传导性聋。

治疗

若无症状则无需治疗。传导性聋者需行听骨链成形术。

Local conditions of the tympanic membrane

Bullous myringitis

Aetiology

An influenza virus infection of the tympanic membrane and deep external meatus, often associated with an acute otitis media.

Clinical features

Presents as otalgia, deafness and serosanguinous otorrhoea. Haemorrhagic bullae are seen on otoscopy (Fig. 21). Secondary bacterial infection can occur with purulent otorrhoea leading to otitis externa.

Management

Treat with analgesics; local and systemic antibiotics for secondary bacterial infection.

Tympanosclerosis

Aetiology

Deposits of collagen beneath the mucosa of the tympanic membrane and middle ear following otitis media or middle ear surgery, particularly grommet insertion.

Clinical features

Tympanosclerosis is mostly asymptomatic. Deposits are visible as white 'chalk patches' in the tympanic membrane (Fig. 22). Middle ear deposits may cause conductive deafness by ossicular fixation.

Management

None if asymptomatic. Ossiculoplasty may be required for conductive deafness.

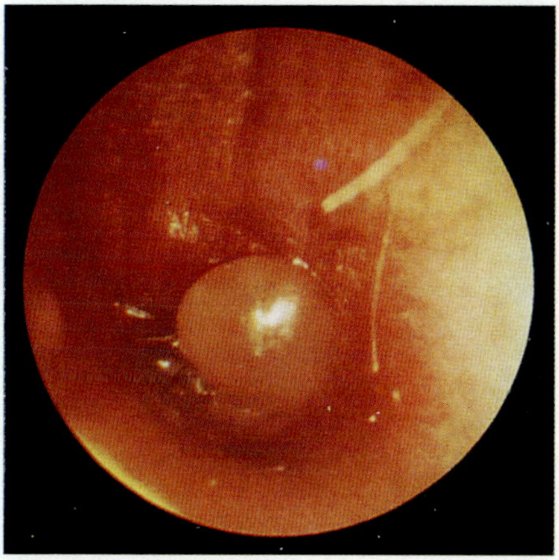

图 21　大疱性鼓膜炎
Bullous myringitis.

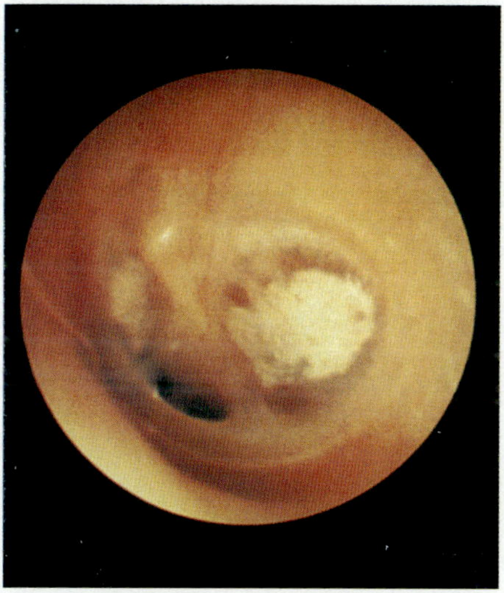

图 22　鼓室硬化的鼓膜表现
Tympanosclerosis of the tympanic membrane.

7 渗出性中耳炎

病因

中耳积液，无论是上呼吸道感染引起的急性发作者，还是儿童期腺样体肥大引起的慢性病程者，常常是由于咽鼓管阻塞所造成的。

成人的中耳积液可能是由于鼻咽部肿物阻塞咽鼓管而形成。飞行或潜水时气压的改变也可以造成中耳积液即耳气压伤。

发病率

中耳积液是儿童的常见病，尤其多见于4～7岁的儿童。

临床特征

耳镜检查鼓膜混浊且光锥消失（图23）。鼓膜上常可见到自锤骨柄呈放射状的小血管，偶尔也可见到液平面（图24）。由于中耳积液引起儿童听力下降，可导致语言发育不良和学习障碍。中耳积液可以通过声阻抗检查来确诊，即检查在外耳道压力变化下鼓膜的顺应性。

治疗

药物治疗：包括局部和全身应用减充血剂。

手术治疗：鼓膜切开术和鼓膜置管术（图25、26）。儿童可能需做腺样体切除术，成人必须除外鼻咽部肿物。

Middle ear effusions

Aetiology

Middle ear effusion is often associated with Eustachian tube obstruction, either acute during upper respiratory infections or chronic as in childhood adenoid hypertrophy. In adults middle ear effusions may result from Eustachian tube obstruction by a nasopharyngeal neoplasm. Changes in atmospheric pressure occurring during flight or diving may also result in effusions: otitic barotrauma.

Incidence

Middle ear effusion is a common paediatric problem, particularly in the 4-7 age group.

Clinical features

On otoscopy the tympanic membrane is dull with a loss of light reflex (Fig. 23). Small vessels are often seen radiating from the handle of the malleus and occasionally a fluid level is seen (Fig. 24). Deafness in children may lead to poor language development and educational performance. Diagnosis may be confirmed by impedance audiometry in which the compliance of the tympanic membrane is measured in response to pressure changes in the external auditory meatus.

Management

Medical treatment: consists of the use of topical and systemic decongestants.
Surgical treatment: consists of myringotomy and insertion of a ventilation tube into the affected tympanic membrane (Figs 25 & 26). Children may also require an adenoidectomy whilst in adults a nasopharyngeal tumour must be excluded.

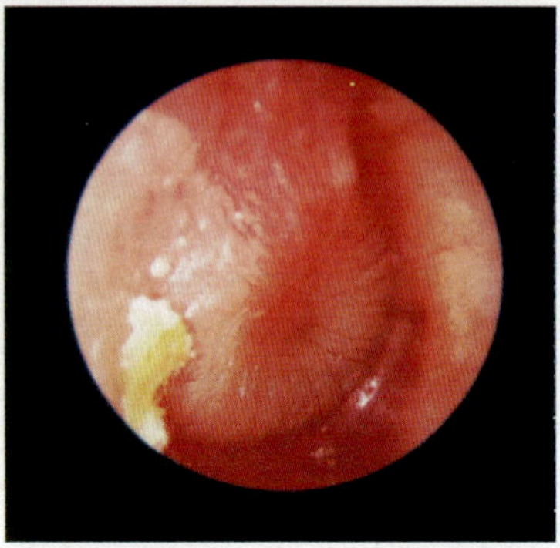

图 23　胶耳
'Glue' ear.

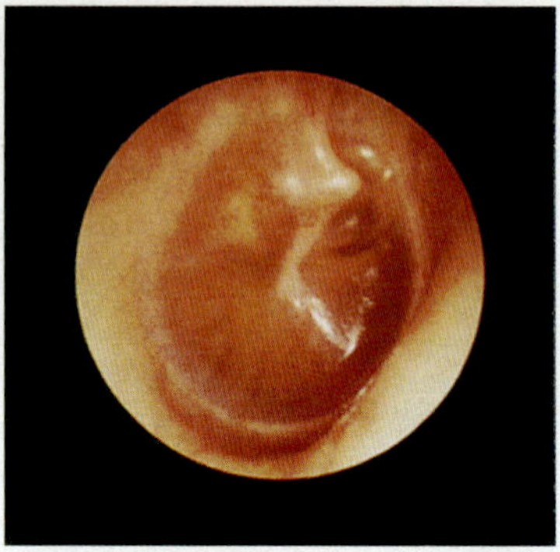

图 24　中耳积液，可见液平面
Serous middle ear effusion with fluid level.

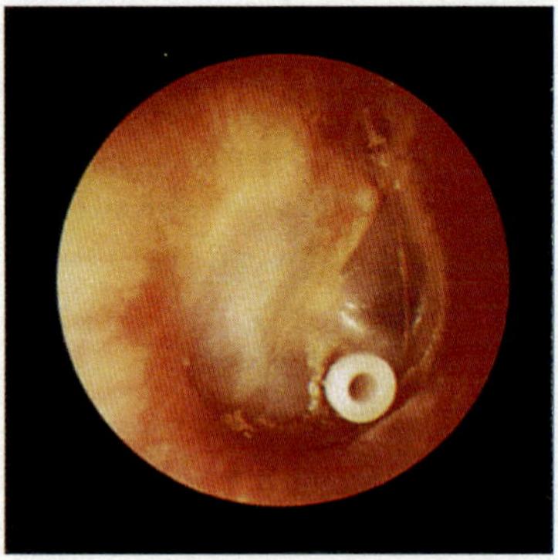

图 25　置入鼓膜的中耳通气管
Grommet in situ.

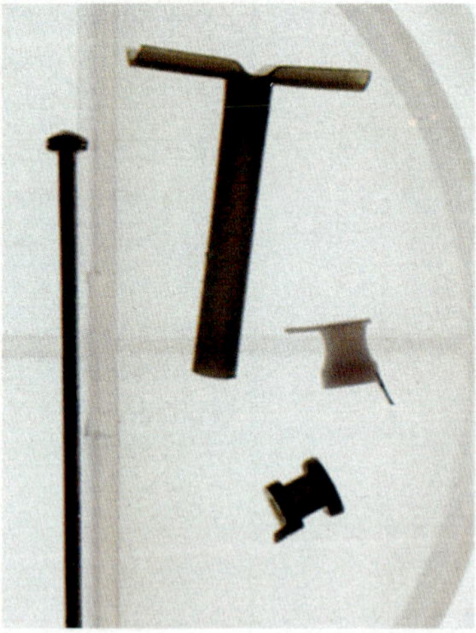

图 26　各种鼓膜通气管：Goode T 型管，Shah 和 Sheppard 通气管（自上而下）
Types of ventilation tube: Goode T tube, Shah and Sheppard grommets (top to bottom).

化脓性中耳炎

急性中耳炎

病因

是中耳腔的急性感染，常见于幼儿。往往是上呼吸道感染的一部分。流感嗜血杆菌和肺炎球菌是最常见的致病菌。

临床特征

表现为严重的耳痛和听力下降。鼓膜充血而膨隆（图27）。鼓膜穿孔后可见脓性的耳溢液。

治疗

口服抗生素（阿莫西林、复方磺胺甲噁唑或红霉素）以及适当的止痛剂。

急性乳突炎

病因

急性乳突炎可以是急性中耳炎的并发症，是乳突气房的急性炎症。

临床特征

表现为耳痛加重，鼓窦区有压痛。外耳道后上壁的水肿可造成耳道变窄。严重者可形成骨膜下脓肿而将患耳推向前方（图28）。CT显示乳突气房增高密度影可确诊此病（图29）。

治疗

静脉注射或肌肉注射大剂量的抗生素。若抗生素治疗无效，或骨膜下脓肿已形成，则需行乳突凿开术以引流脓液。

Suppurative otitis media

Acute otitis media

Aetiology

Acute infection of the middle ear cleft, common in young children. This usually occurs as part of an upper respiratory tract infection, with *Haemophilus influenzae* and *Pneumococcus* being the most common pathogens.

Clinical features

Presents as severe otalgia and deafness. The tympanic membrane is red and bulging (Fig. 27). Rupture may occur leading to purulent otorrhoea.

Management

Treat with oral antibiotic therapy (amoxicillin, co-trimoxazole or erythromycin) and adequate analgesia.

Acute mastoiditis

Aetiology

Acute mastoiditis may complicate acute otitis media. Infection of the mastoid air cell system occurs.

Clinical features

Presents as worsening of otalgia with tenderness over the mastoid antrum. The external meatus may be narrowed by oedema of the posterior-superior wall. In advanced cases a subperiosteal abscess may push the ear forward (Fig. 28). Diagnosis is confirmed by opacity of the mastoid cells on CT scan (Fig. 29).

Management

Initially high-dose parenteral antibiotic therapy is required, although in cases that fail to respond to antibiotics, or in which a subperiosteal abscess has formed, surgical drainage via a cortical mastoidectomy is required.

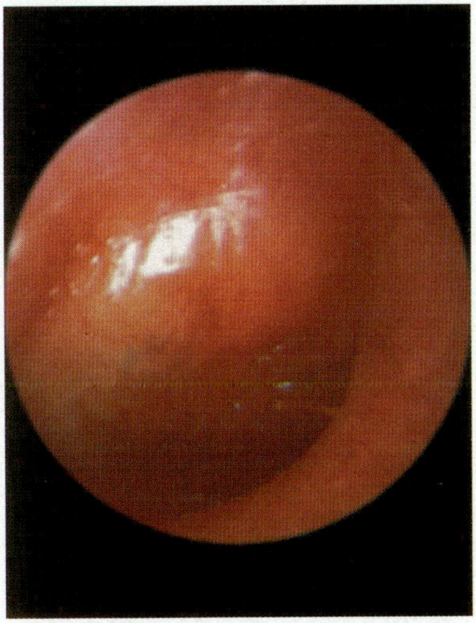

图 27　急性中耳炎
Acute otitis media.

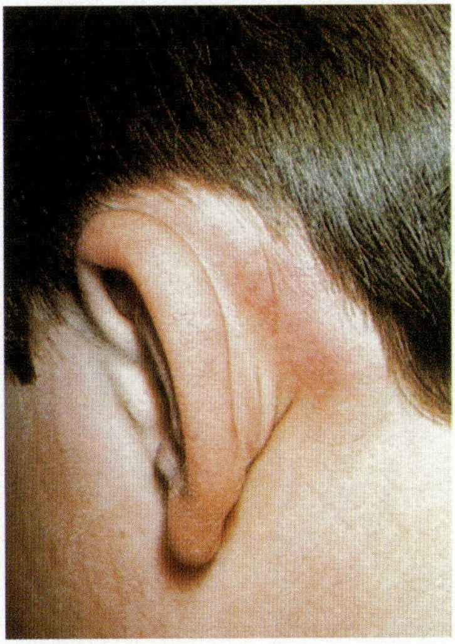

图 28　急性乳突炎，可见耳后肿胀、充血
Postauricular swelling and redness in acute mastoiditis.

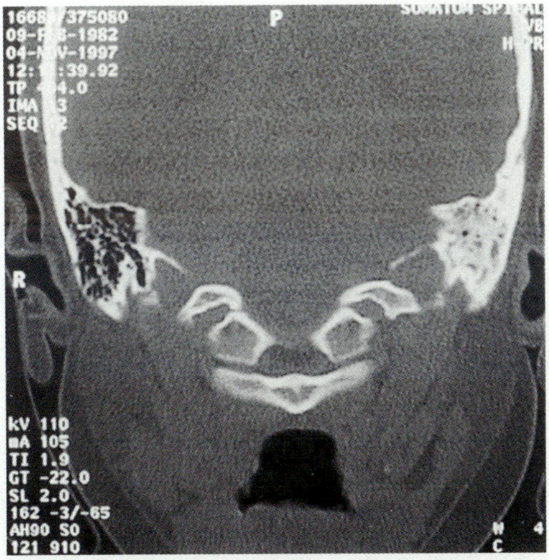

图 29　CT 显示乳突炎时乳突区增高密度影
CT scan showing mastoid opacity in mastoiditis.

慢性中耳炎

病因

中耳腔的慢性炎症常与鼓膜穿孔相联系。鼓膜穿孔可以是既往急性中耳炎所致的鼓膜穿孔未能愈合，也可因直接或间接的创伤而造成。在儿童，中耳置管脱出后鼓膜穿孔可持续存在。致病菌可以通过咽鼓管或外耳道进入中耳腔。慢性中耳炎也常导致听骨链的破坏，砧镫关节是最常见的受累部位。

临床特征

表现为鼓膜紧张部中央型穿孔（图 30、31）、反复耳流脓及传导性耳聋。这种类型的穿孔被认为是“安全的”，因为很少引起神经系统的并发症。上鼓室或边缘型穿孔（图 32）常常与胆脂瘤的形成有关，被认为是“危险的”。

治疗

对于中央型穿孔应该保持其干燥。如果反复发生耳流脓，应该使用含激素和抗生素的滴耳液，而且应该注意鼻咽部、鼻腔和鼻旁窦有无潜在的感染灶。可采取鼓膜成形术来修补干性穿孔。外伤性鼓膜穿孔可自行愈合。

Chronic otitis media

Aetiology

Chronic inflammation of the middle ear cleft is usually associated with a perforation of the tympanic membrane. Perforations usually result from previous episodes of acute otitis media when the membrane fails to heal following rupture, but can be due to direct or indirect trauma. In children, perforations can persist following extrusion of ventilation tubes from the tympanic membrane. Organisms can reach the middle ear from the Eustachian tube or from the external meatus. Chronic middle ear infection is also associated with ossicular damage, with the incudostapedial joint being the most commonly affected linkage.

Clinical features

A central perforation in the pars tensa part of the membrane (Figs 30 & 31) is associated with recurrent otorrhoea and conductive deafness. This type of perforation is regarded as 'safe' as neurological complications are rare. An attic or marginal perforation (Fig. 32) can be associated with the development of a cholesteatoma and is regarded as 'unsafe'.

Management

Cases of central perforation should be kept dry. If recurrent otorrhoea occurs, ear drops containing a mixture of steroid and antibiotic are used and attention should be paid to possible sources of infection in the nasopharynx, nose and paranasal sinuses. A dry perforation can be repaired by myringoplasty. Traumatic central perforations usually heal spontaneously.

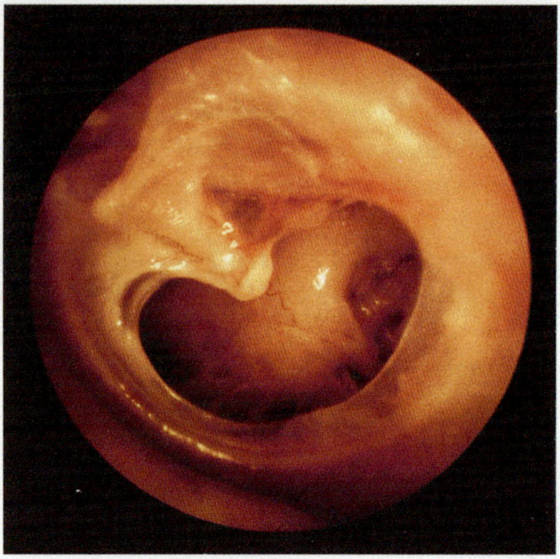

图 30　干性中央型穿孔
Dry central perforation.

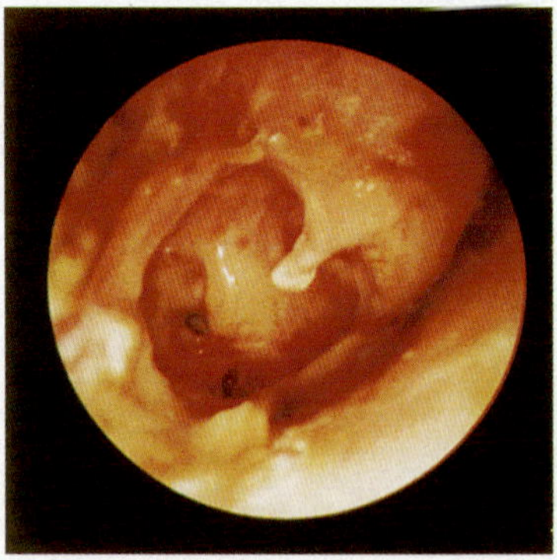

图 31　次全穿孔
Subtotal perforation.

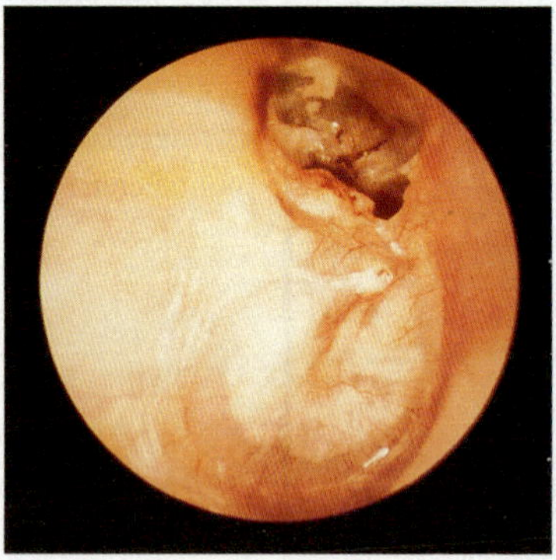

图 32　干性上鼓室穿孔
Dry attic perforation.

胆脂瘤

是位于中耳或乳突腔内的角质化的复层鳞状上皮球，可以增大并破坏或侵蚀局部结构。这是危险型慢性中耳疾病的一个特征。

病因

关于胆脂瘤形成的最广为人接受的学说是上皮移入－袋状内陷学说。当咽鼓管阻塞，中耳形成负压，鼓膜就发生了内陷，内陷通常发生在上鼓室。鼓膜上皮正常的脱屑聚集在内陷所形成的囊袋里。不断增大的内陷袋形成了胆脂瘤。先天性胆脂瘤非常少见（图 33），是由先天残留在颞骨的鳞状上皮所引起的。

临床特征

表现为进行性的传导性听力下降，以及脓性的伴有恶臭的耳溢液。骨质破坏可引起疼痛或眩晕。耳镜检查可见上鼓室部位的内陷袋或穿孔（图 34），或者在鼓膜后部边缘处见到片状的白色脱屑。应注意患者有无眼震或神经系统受累的其他表现。

治疗

行乳突根治术，包括清除胆脂瘤、中耳内的结构及骨性外耳道后壁，形成一光滑的、向外耳道开放的乳突腔，便于术后观察。改良乳突根治术可保留听力，包括听骨链重建和修复鼓膜等（图 35）。

9 Cholesteatoma

A ball of keratinizing stratified squamous epithelium in the middle ear cleft or mastoid which enlarges and can destroy or erode local structures. It is a feature of the 'unsafe' type of chronic middle ear disease.

Aetiology

The most widely accepted theory of its development is the immigration-retraction pocket theory: in response to Eustachian tube obstruction and negative middle ear pressure an inward retraction of the tympanic membrane occurs, usually in the attic region. Desquamated epithelium normally shed from the membrane into the meatus collects in the pocket, the continued enlargement of which results in the formation of a cholesteatoma sac. Congenital cholesteatoma is very rare (Fig.33) and results from congenital squamous cell rests within the temporal bone.

Clinical features

Presents as progressive conductive hearing loss with purulent, and often offensive, otorrhoea. Pain or vertigo due to bony erosion may also occur. Otoscopy reveals a retraction pocket or perforation in the attic or posterior marginal region of the tympanic membrane (Fig.34) with flaky white debris visible in the defect. Nystagmus and other evidence of neurological involvement should be sought.

Management

Radical mastoidectomy involves removal of the cholesteatoma, middle ear structures and bone of the bony external meatus, producing a smooth exteriorized mastoid cavity accessible for inspection. The operation may be modified in order to conserve hearing by retaining part of the ossicular chain and tympanic membrane (Fig. 35).

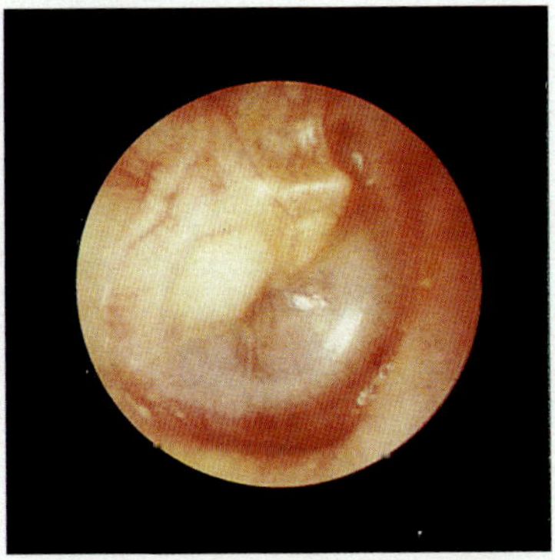

图 33　先天性胆脂瘤，隐藏在完整的鼓膜里面
Congenital cholesteatoma behind an intact tympanic membrane.

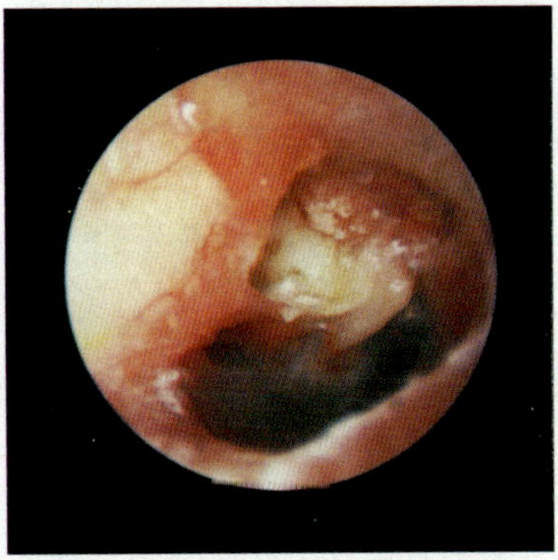

图 34　上鼓室穿孔以及胆脂瘤
Attic perforation with cholesteatoma.

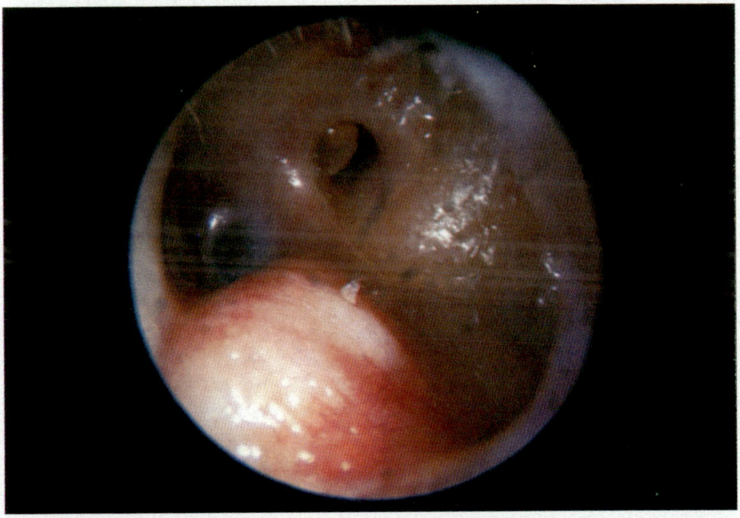

图 35　已经愈合的左侧改良乳突根治术后的术腔
Healed left modified radical mastoidectomy cavity.

化脓性中耳炎的并发症

颅外并发症

面神经麻痹

病因	中耳或乳突内的胆脂瘤压迫面神经所致。
临床特征	表现为部分或全部的周围性面瘫（图 36），耳镜检查确认患有慢性中耳疾病。
治疗	立即行乳突开放的面神经减压术。

化脓性迷路炎

病因	骨迷路被破坏所致，最常见于外半规管。早期，通过加压于外耳道内的空气可机械性地刺激迷路引起眩晕（瘘管试验）。晚期，内耳的化脓性感染导致严重的眩晕和感音神经性聋。
治疗	静脉给予抗生素，行乳突手术，清除胆脂瘤。

岩尖综合征（Gradenigo 综合征）

表现为耳溢液、眼球深部的疼痛和复视。这是由于岩尖部气房的感染引起的第五和第六脑神经受刺激所致（图 37）。

Complications of suppurative otitis media

Extracranial

Facial nerve paralysis

Aetiology

Pressure by cholesteatoma on the facial nerve in the middle ear or mastoid.

Clinical features

Presents as partial or complete lower motor neurone facial paralysis (Fig. 36) with evidence of chronic middle ear disease on otoscopy.

Management

Treatment is by immediate surgical decompression of the facial nerve via a mastoidectomy operation.

Suppurative labyrinthitis

Aetiology

Follows erosion of the bony labyrinth most commonly over the lateral semicircular canal. In the early stages compression of the air in the external meatus causes vertigo from mechanical stimulation of the labyrinth (fistula test). Later purulent infection in the inner ear causes severe vertigo and sensorineural deafness.

Management

Treatment is by intravenous antibiotics and eradication of cholesteatoma via mastoidectomy.

Gradenigo's syndrome

Otorrhoea is associated with pain behind the eye and diplopia, caused by fifth and sixth nerve irritation resulting from air cell infection at the petrous apex (Fig. 37).

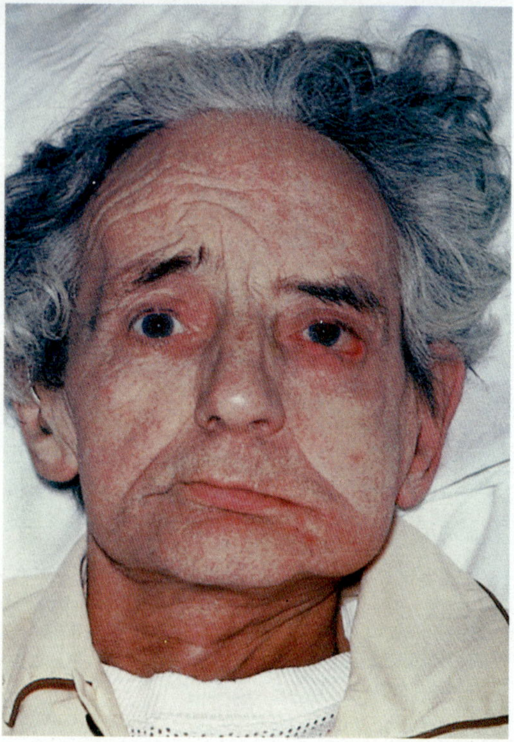

图 36　完全的周围性面瘫
Complete lower motor neurone facial palsy.

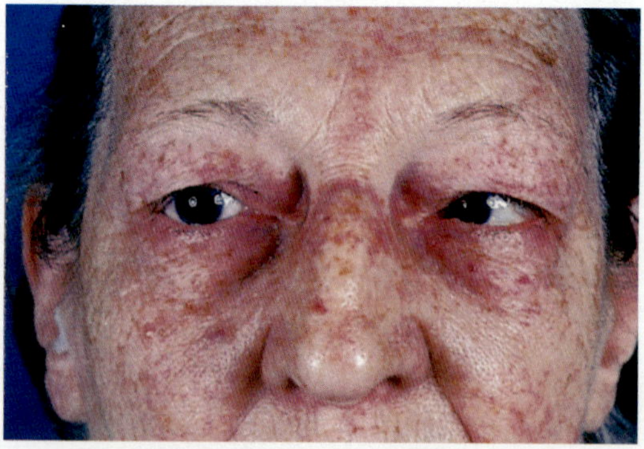

图 37　岩尖综合征：患者右斜视
Gradenigo's syndrome: patient looking to right.

颅内并发症

致病菌可经由中耳通过血栓性静脉炎或直接穿过中颅窝或后颅窝的脑膜，造成颅内扩散。

脑膜炎

临床特征 表现为头痛、颈强直和畏光。行腰椎穿刺检查可以确诊。肺炎球菌和流感嗜血杆菌为常见的致病菌。

治疗 静脉给予抗生素。一旦脑膜炎得以控制，即行乳突凿开术。

乙状窦血栓性静脉炎

中耳和乳突的感染经骨壁累及乙状窦。

临床特征 表现为头痛、发热和僵直。血栓扩展至上矢状窦可导致脑脊液流出道梗阻，引起耳源性脑积水。

治疗 包括静脉给予抗生素及乳突凿开术，术中应将感染的血栓自窦腔中清除（图 38）。

颅内脓肿

可发生硬膜外、硬膜下及脑脓肿。感染扩展至中和后颅窝可分别导致颞叶和小脑脓肿。可通过 CT 检查确诊（图 39、40）。治疗需神经外科医生行脓肿引流。

Intracranial

Intracranial spread of organisms may occur via the middle ear by thrombophlebitis or by penetration of the dura of the middle or posterior cranial fossae.

Meningitis

Clinical features

Presents as headache, neck stiffness and photophobia. Lumbar puncture confirms the diagnosis. *Pneumococcus* and *Haemophilus influenzae* are common pathogens.

Management

Treatment is by intravenous antibiotics followed by mastoidectomy once the meningitis has resolved.

Venous sinus thrombosis

Follows spread of middle ear and mastoid infection through the bone over the sigmoid sinus.

Clinical features

Presents as headache, pyrexia and rigors. Extension of thrombus to the superior sagittal sinus leads to CSF outflow obstruction: otitic hydrocephalus.

Management

Treatment is by intravenous antibiotics and mastoidectomy, during which infected thrombus may need to be removed from the sinus lumen (Fig. 38).

Intracranial abscess

Extradural, subdural and cerebral abscesses occur. Infection spreads into the middle and posterior cranial fossae leading to temporal lobe and cerebellar abscesses respectively. Diagnosis is by CT scan (Figs 39 & 40) and treatment by neurosurgical drainage.

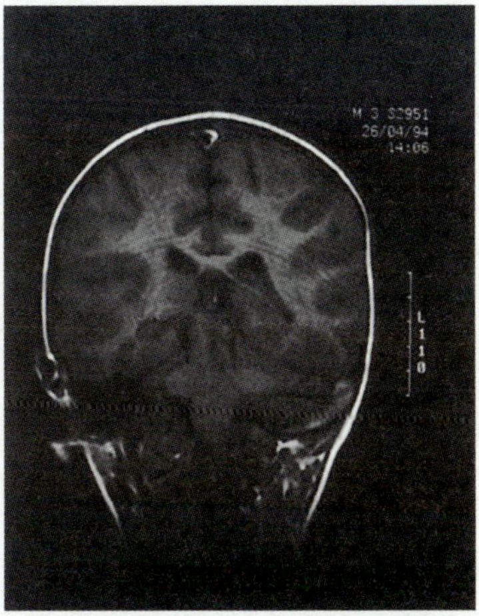

图 38　乙状窦血栓形成（MRI）
Lateral sinus thrombosis (MRI).

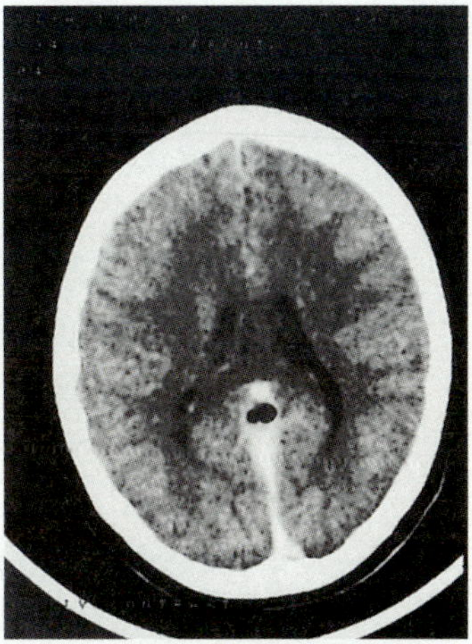

图 39　CT 显示硬膜下脓肿，其间可见空气
CT scan showing air in the subdural space in a subdural abscess.

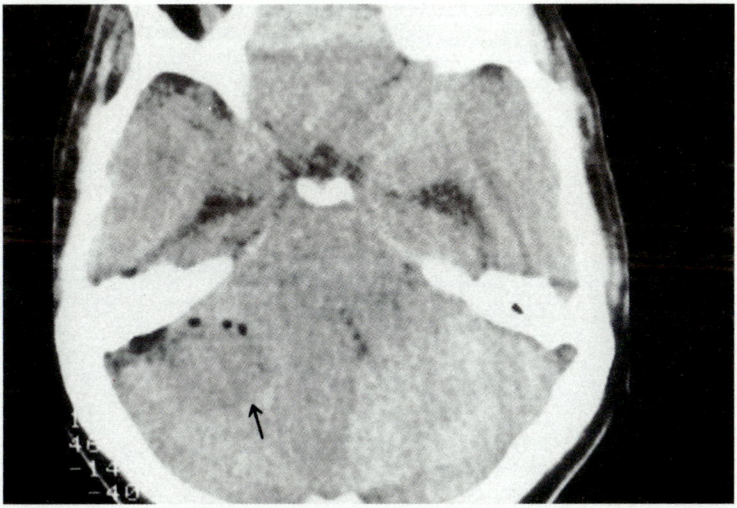

图 40　CT 显示耳源性小脑脓肿
Otogenic cerebellar abscess on CT scan.

11 耳硬化症

原发于听泡骨质的疾病，引起传导性聋，常由于镫骨固定引起。晚期可发生感音神经性聋。

发病率

通常是双侧发病，常见于15至45岁的人群。患者常有耳鸣，25%的患者有位置性眩晕，70%的患者有家族史。

临床特征

鼓膜外观通常是正常的。鼓膜呈粉红色的现象（即Schwartze征）很少见，若出现则表示疾病呈活动状态（图41）。早期纯音测听检查显示传导性聋，常在2000Hz处见到Cahart切迹（图42）。

治疗

对耳硬化症的患者来说气导助听器常常很有效。在镫骨足板造孔手术中，镫骨弓被活塞所取代，活塞常由聚四氟乙烯树脂制成（图43）。行镫骨足板造孔术可使大多数患者听力显著提高，但偶尔也可引起重度耳聋及眩晕等并发症。

极少数的患者合并成骨不全（van der Hoeve 综合征），这些患者具有蓝色的巩膜，不难辨认。对此类患者行镫骨足板切除术很少奏效。

Otosclerosis

A disease primarily of the bone of the otic capsule which causes a conductive hearing loss, usually because of stapes fixation. A sensorineural deafness may occur in the later stages.

Incidence

The disease is usually bilateral and presents between the ages of 15 and 45 years. Tinnitus is common and 25% of patients have positional vertigo. 70% have a family history of otosclerosis.

Clinical features

Examination of the tympanic membrane is usually normal, the pink drum (Schwartze sign) being rare and indicative of active disease (Fig. 41). In the early stages the audiogram shows a pure conductive loss, frequently with a Cahart's notch at 2000Hz (Fig. 42).

Management

An air conduction hearing aid is frequently very successful for the patient. In the stapedotomy operation the stapes arch is replaced by a piston, usually made of Teflon (Fig. 43). Stapedotomy will produce excellent improvement in hearing level in the majority of cases, although profound deafness and vertigo are occasional complications.

A rare variant is seen in association with osteogenesis imperfecta (van der Hoeve syndrome), these patients being recognized by their blue sclera. Stapedectomy is less successful in these cases.

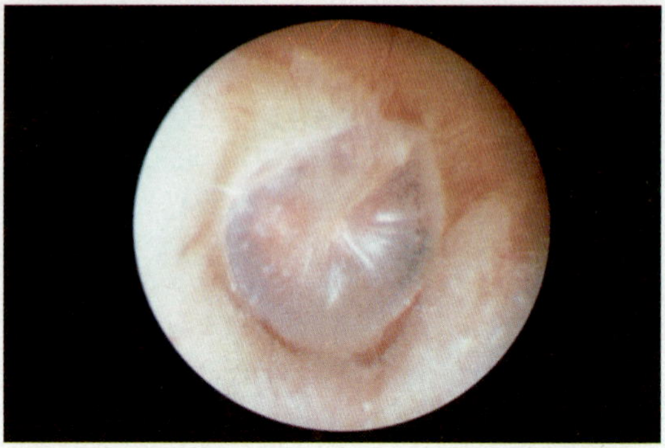

图 41　Schwartze 征：鼓膜后方火烈鸟样的粉红色
Schwartze sign: flamingo pink flush behind tympanic membrane.

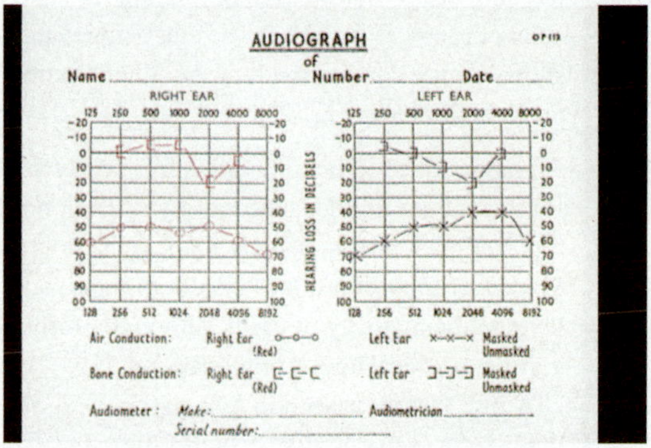

图 42　纯音测听检查显示双侧 Cahart 切迹
Pure tone audiogram with bilateral Cahart's notches.

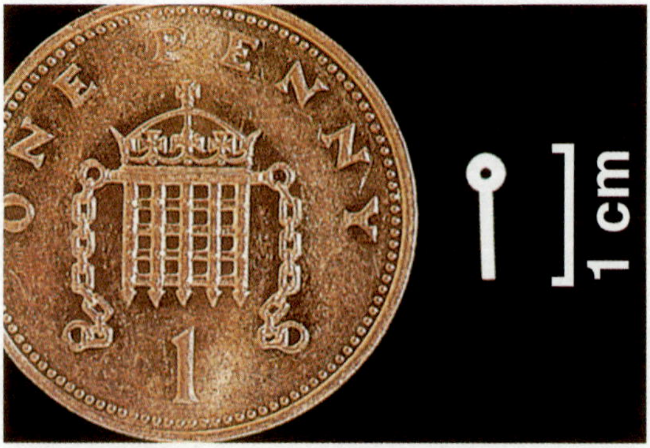

图 43　聚四氟乙烯树脂制成的镫骨假体
Teflon stapes prosthesis.

鼓膜成形术（鼓膜修补术）

中央型穿孔当伴有耳聋或反复中耳感染，或因游泳、应聘等情况需要完整的鼓膜时，可以行鼓膜成形术。经常采用颞肌表面的筋膜来修补鼓膜（图 44），可以用外植法或内植法。

听骨链成形术

由于慢性炎症、创伤或先天畸形所引起的听骨链中断而造成的传导性耳聋可行听骨链重建术。听骨的赝复物可以是自体的，也可以是合成材料。骨质是一种不错的材料，可能的情况下可以用患者残余的砧骨，将其重新塑形再重建听骨链。

清除乳突病变：乳突切除术

急性乳突炎在大剂量抗生素治疗无效后，慢性乳突炎致耳漏，以及中耳、乳突胆脂瘤者需行乳突根治术。

经皮质乳突切除术：指清除乳突气房，但不涉及外耳道、听小骨及鼓膜的手术（图 45）。

乳突根治术及改良乳突根治术：为清理胆脂瘤施行的手术，指去除外耳道后壁骨质，形成一大的术腔，此种术腔也便于术后清理（图 46）。

Middle ear microsurgery

Myringoplasty

Central perforations may be repaired when accompanied by deafness or recurrent middle ear infections, or when an intact tympanic membrane is required for swimming, or as a condition of employment. Fascia overlying the temporalis muscle is usually used (Fig. 44) and may be placed medial (underlay) or lateral (onlay) to the perforation.

Ossiculoplasty

Performed for conductive deafness where the ossicular chain has been interrupted by chronic infection, trauma or congenital deformity. Replacement ossicles may be constructed from natural or synthetic materials. Bone is the favoured material; where possible the patient's own incus remnant is remodelled and transposed.

Eradication of mastoid disease: mastoidectomy

Performed for acute mastoiditis failing to respond to high-dose antibiotics, otorrhoea due to chronic mastoid infection, and middle ear and mastoid cholesteatoma.

Cortical mastoidectomy: involves exenterating the mastoid air cell system without interfering with the external meatus, ossicles or tympanic membrane (Fig. 45).

Radical and modified radical mastoidectomy: for cholesteatoma involves removal of the posterior meatal wall, creating a large cavity accessible for cleaning (Fig. 46).

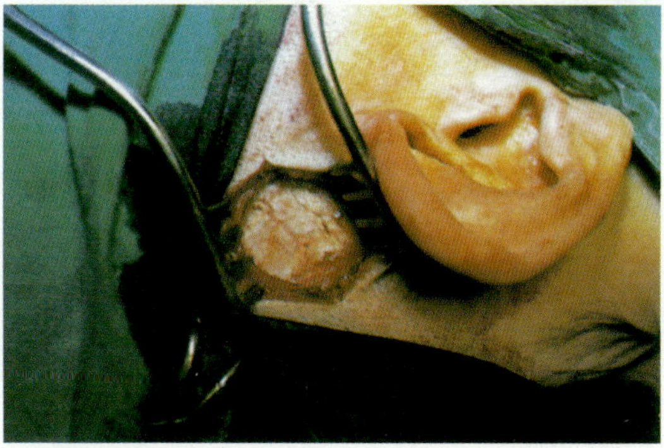

图 44　取颞肌筋膜移植物
Harvesting a temporalis fascia graft.

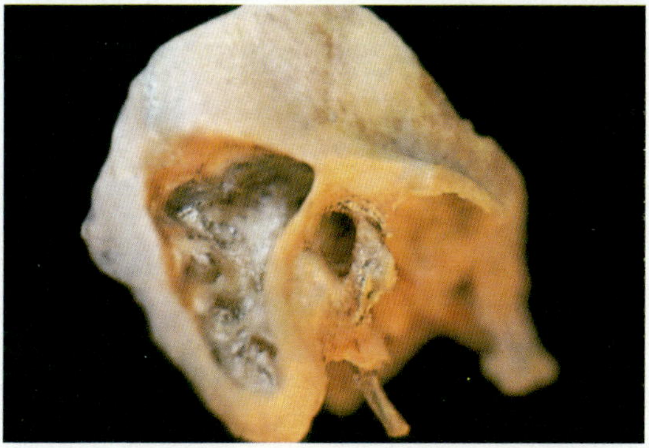

图 45　经皮质乳突切除术（尸头解剖标本）
Cortical mastoidectomy (cadaver dissection).

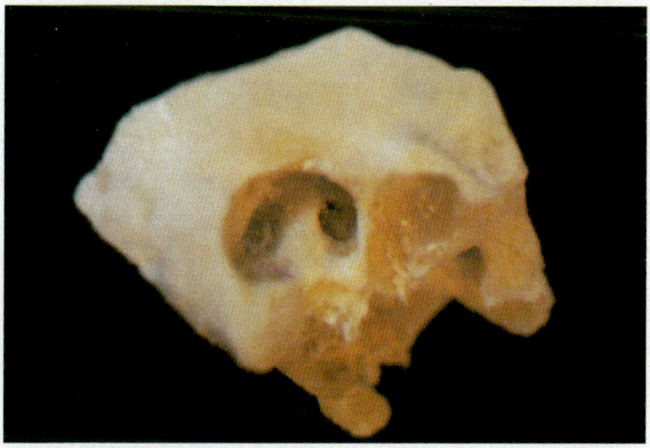

图 46　乳突根治术（尸头解剖标本）
Radical mastoidectomy (cadaver dissection).

13 面神经麻痹

从脑干面神经核至面肌之间任何一处的面神经中断都可造成周围性面神经麻痹（面瘫）。

Bell 面瘫（特发性）

临床特征

是最常见的周围性面瘫，没有明确的病因。病毒感染和血管因素是较普遍的病因假说。可表现为部分或完全性面瘫。

治疗

90% 的患者可以完全恢复。激素应用和手术减压对该病的治疗效果尚存争议。

耳部带状疱疹（Ramsay Hunt 综合征）

临床特征

带状疱疹病毒侵及面神经，鼓膜、耳廓或腭部可见疱疹（图 47、48）。可仅表现为严重的耳痛，亦可累及听神经及三叉神经。

治疗

60% 的患者可以完全康复。如果尽早给予抗病毒药物阿昔洛韦，可以促进患者恢复。应用激素或行面神经减压术对该病的治疗价值尚未得到证实。

颞骨骨折

临床特征

纵行骨折者（占颞骨骨折的 80%）中约 20% 出现面瘫及传导性聋。横行骨折者（占颞骨骨折的 20%）中约 50% 出现面瘫及感音神经性聋。通过CT检查可以确诊（图 49）。

治疗

对于立即出现的、完全性面瘫应行面神经检查术，但术后可能出现耳聋。

Facial nerve palsy 13

Disruption of the lower motor neurone facial nerve can occur at any point between its brainstem nucleus and the facial musculature.

Bell's (idiopathic) palsy

Clinical features Most common palsy with no identifiable cause although a viral or vascular aetiology postulated. Palsy may be partial or complete.

Management Total recovery occurs in 90% of cases. Treatment with steroids or surgical decompression controversial.

Ramsay Hunt syndrome

Clinical features Herpes zoster involvement of the facial nerve with herpetic vesicles on the tympanic membrane (Fig. 47), pinna (Fig. 48) or palate. May present with severe otalgia alone. Auditory and trigeminal nerves may be affected.

Management Recovers fully in about 60% of cases. If given early, the antiviral agent aciclovir may enhance recovery. The value of steroids or surgical decompression of the nerve remains unproven.

Temporal bone fracture

Clinical features Longitudinal fractures (80%) are associated with a facial palsy in 20% of cases and a conductive deafness. Transverse fractures (20%) are associated with a facial palsy in 50% of cases and a sensorineural deafness. Diagnosis is confirmed by CT scan (Fig. 49).

Management Exploration of the nerve may be indicated in cases of immediate, complete paralysis but is likely to be followed by deafness.

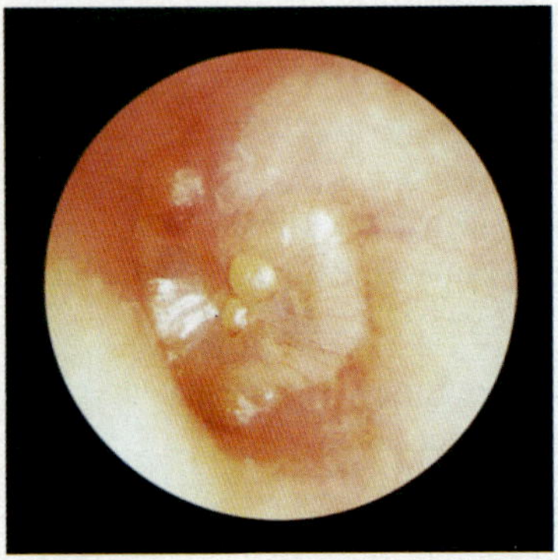

图 47　鼓膜上的疱疹
Herpetic vesicles on the tympanic membrane.

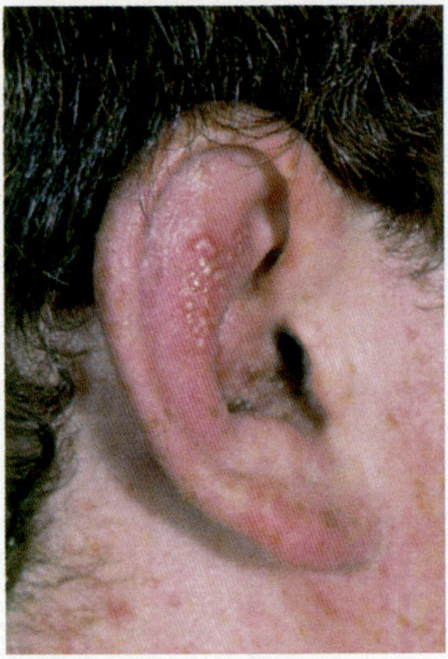

图 48　耳廓上的疱疹
Herpetic vesicles on the pinna.

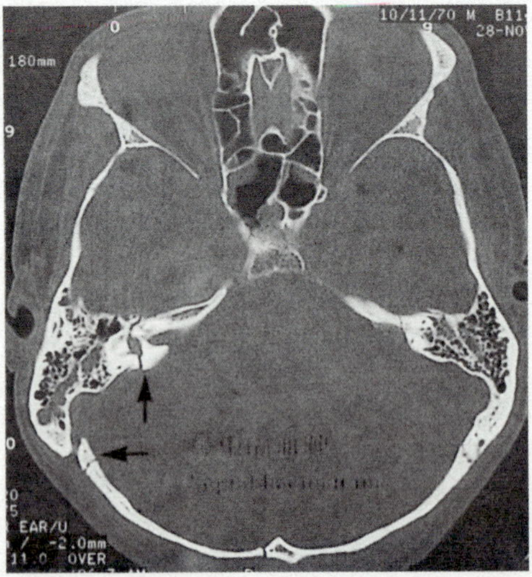

图 49　颞骨骨折
Temporal bone fracture.

耳源性眩晕

耳源性眩晕是对运动的一种幻觉或错觉。影响前庭器官的疾病可以产生旋转性眩晕伴随水平性眼震。

检查

冷热水试验（图 50）：通过向外耳道内注入不同温度的水来刺激前庭器官，记录诱发眼震持续的时间，然后对双侧反应进行比较。

位置性眼震检查（图 51）：通过头位的变动来激发眩晕（位置性眩晕）。这可能是内耳疾病、颈椎关节强直或影响到脑干前庭中枢的疾病的一个特征。

梅尼埃病

病因

不明。可能是由于内耳内淋巴生成与吸收的不平衡引起，或内耳免疫功能紊乱所造成。

临床特征

表现为反复发作的旋转性眩晕、耳鸣和感音神经性聋。早期为单侧发病。

治疗

急性发作时可用前庭镇静剂。手术可为保守性（内淋巴囊减压术）或破坏性手术（迷路切除术或前庭神经切断术）。鼓室内注射庆大霉素也可做为治疗方案之一。

突发性单侧前庭功能丧失

病因

不明。有关的假说有病毒感染、缺血和内耳膜破裂。

临床特征

表现为突然发生的眩晕。当中枢代偿以后，眩晕得以缓解。

治疗

急性发作期用前庭镇静剂。

引起眩晕的其他原因有梅毒、化脓性迷路炎、颞骨骨折和耳毒性药物。

14 Otogenic vertigo

Otogenic vertigo is an hallucination or a false sensation of movement. Disease affecting the vestibular apparatus may produce rotatory vertigo accompanied by horizontal nystagmus.

Testing

Caloric testing (Fig. 50).Involves stimulating the vestibular apparatus by irrigating the external meatus with water at varying temperatures; the duration of induced nystagmus is recorded, allowing comparison between the two sides.

Positional testing (Fig. 51).Vertigo provoked by head movements (positional vertigo) may be a feature of inner ear disease, cervical spondylosis or disease affecting central vestibular pathways in the brainstem.

Ménière's disease

Aetiology

Unknown; may be due to imbalance between production and absorption of inner ear endolymph or disturbance of inner ear immunity.

Clinical features

Episodic rotatory vertigo, tinnitus and sensorineural deafness may be present. Unilateral in early stages.

Management

Vestibular sedatives for acute attacks. Surgery may be conservative (endolymphatic sac decompression) or destructive (labyrinthectomy or vestibular neurectomy). Intratympanic gentamicin is also an option.

Sudden unilateral vestibular failure

Aetiology

Unknown aetiology. Viral infection, ischaemia and inner ear membrane rupture have been postulated.

Clinical features

Presents with sudden onset of vertigo. Recovery takes place by central compensation.

Management

Vestibular sedatives are useful in the acute phase.

Other causes of vertigo are syphilis, suppurative labyrinthitis, temporal fractures and ototoxic drugs.

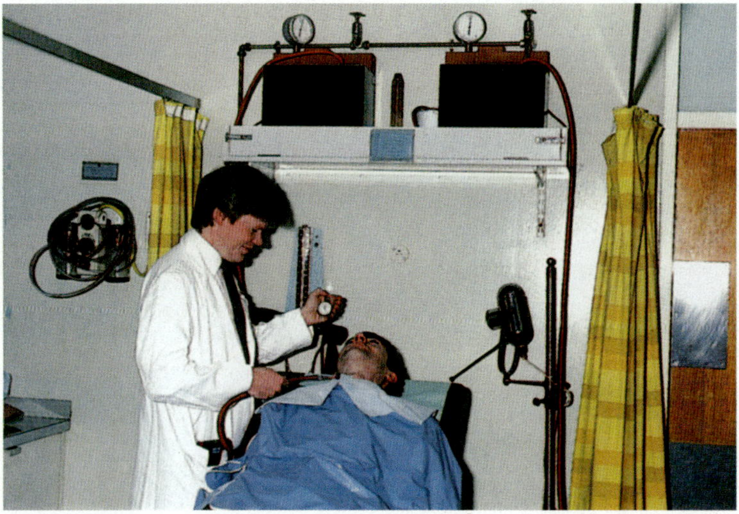

图 50 冷热水试验
Caloric testing.

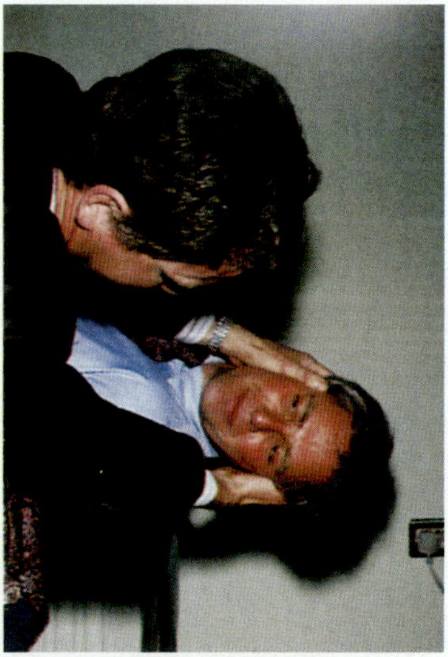

图 51 位置性眼震检查
Positional testing.

15 感音神经性聋

感音神经性聋是耳蜗或其与中枢神经之间的联系出现病变而造成的。该病可以是先天性的（图 52），也可以是后天性的。

先天性

病因

发育不全：内耳部分或完全发育不良。如：Schiebe畸形。

功能缺陷：在解剖上内耳已经发育了，但是神经通路发育不完善。如：Pendred，Hurler 和 Alport 综合征。

宫内/围生期损害：包括缺氧、核黄疸、风疹、巨细胞病毒感染、梅毒、服用沙利度胺等。

后天性

病因

1. 老年性聋：最常见
2. 噪声性聋
3. 梅尼埃病
4. 听神经瘤（图 53）
5. 外伤，如：头部外伤，中耳手术
6. 突发性感音神经性聋
7. 药物性聋，如：庆大霉素（图 54）
8. 梅毒 / 雅司病。

治疗

当所有有效治疗措施应用后，任何类型的感音神经性聋的治疗均需听力康复训练。对于严重耳聋的孩子来说，特殊教育是非常需要的。

Sensorineural hearing loss

Sensorineural hearing loss results from disease in the cochlea or its central neuronal connections. The disease can be congenital (Fig. 52) or acquired.

Congenital

Aetiology

Aplasias. Partial or complete failure of inner ear development, e.g. Schiebe anomaly.

Abiotrophies. Inner ear anatomically developed but neural pathways degenerate prematurely, e.g. Pendred, Hurler and Alport syndromes.

Intrauterine/perinatal damage. Includes hypoxia, kernicterus, rubella, cytomegalovirus, syphilis, thalidomide.

Acquired

Aetiology

- Age-related presbyacusis: the most common
- Noise-induced hearing loss
- Ménière's disease
- Acoustic neuroma (Fig. 53)
- Trauma, e.g. head injury, middle ear surgery
- Sudden (idiopathic) sensorineural hearing loss
- Drug-induced hearing loss, e.g. gentamicin (Fig. 54)
- Syphilis/yaws.

Management

The management of any sensorineural hearing loss involves rehabilitation, once any treatable cause has been excluded. Special schooling may be necessary for the severely deaf child.

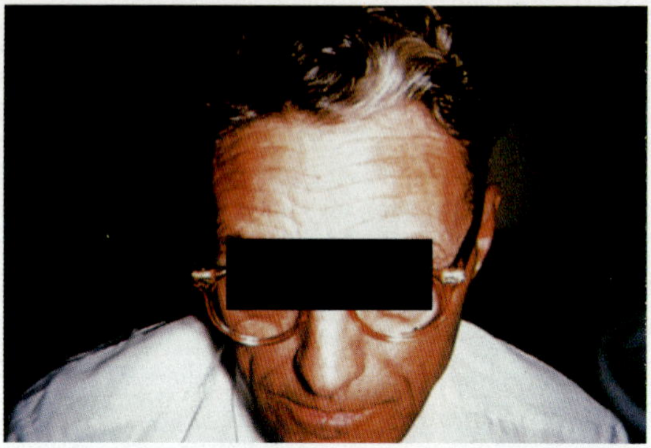

图 52　Waardenburg 综合征：可见白色的额发
White forelock in Waardenburg syndrome.

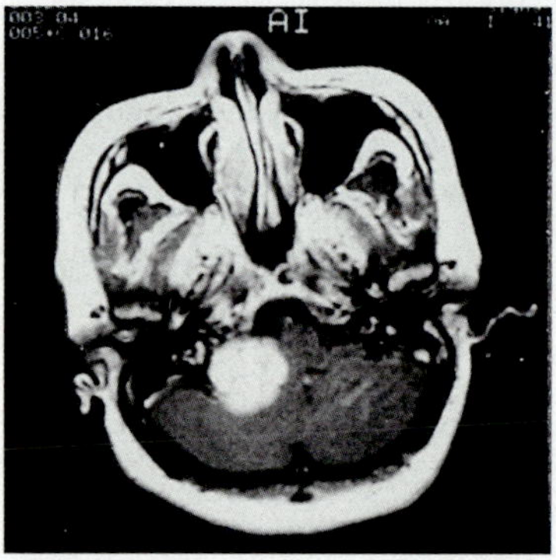

图 53　MRI 检查示后颅窝的听神经瘤
Posterior fossa MRI scan showing an acoustic neuroma.

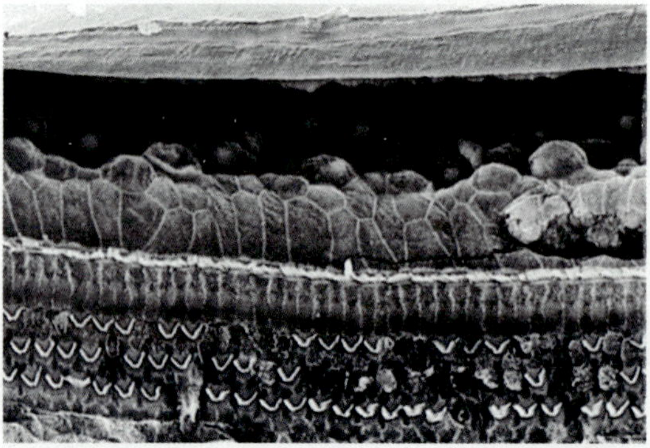

图 54　扫描电镜示庆大霉素损害的耳蜗毛细胞
Scanning electron micrograph of gentamicin-damaged cochlear hair cells.

耳聋的治疗与康复

耳聋的早期诊断是听力康复得以成功的关键，尤其是对于先天性聋的患儿。大部分儿童如果早期能够得到听力的强化训练，那么将拥有口语交流的能力。唇读可以辅助口语交流。严重耳聋的患者可用手语进行交流。

助听器

助听器将传入的声音进行放大及修饰。最先进的助听器应用数字技术使助听器能够适合每个耳聋患者不同程度的听力损失。耳背式助听器（图 55）是最为广泛应用的助听器，另外还有体佩式助听器、耳内式助听器（图 56）。借助于电声放大“回路”系统，助听器可在不同的环境中发挥作用，如剧院或会议大厅。

电子耳蜗

电子耳蜗就是将传入的声波转化为耳蜗部位的直接的电刺激冲动。电极可以放置在耳蜗的表面（耳蜗外）或插入耳蜗腔内（耳蜗内）（图 57）。

电子耳蜗被应用于先天性或后天性严重的感音神经性聋患者。重度聋儿最好在学龄前就植入电子耳蜗。

16 Rehabilitation of deafness

Early diagnosis of deafness is the key to successful auditory rehabilitation, particularly in children with congenital deafness. With early intensive auditory training most children will develop the ability to communicate orally. Lip reading is an adjunct to oral communication. Manual communication, as in sign language, may be applicable for severely deaf people.

Hearing aids

Hearing aids amplify and modify incoming sound. The most modern aids use digital technology to tailor the performance of the aid to individual patterns of hearing loss. The postaural aid (Fig. 55) is most widely used, although body-worn and 'in the ear' alternatives exist (Fig. 56). Aids to communication such as electromagnetic 'loop' systems can enable hearing aids to function in a group environment such as a theatre or lecture hall.

Cochlear implants

Direct electrical stimulation of the cochlear portion of the inner ear in response to incoming sound waves has been investigated in the development of cochlear implants. Electrodes are either placed on the surface of the cochlea (extracochlear) or inserted into the lumen of the cochlea (intracochlear) (Fig. 57).

The use of cochlear implantation is now established in patients with both acquired and congenital severe sensorineural hearing loss. Profoundly deaf children ideally have implants fitted before primary school age.

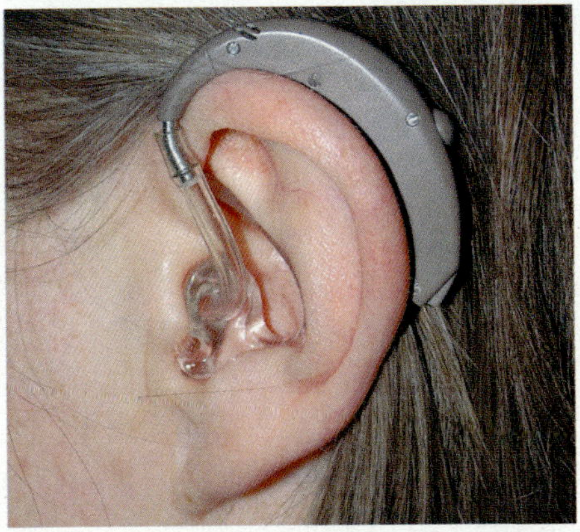

图 55　耳背式助听器
Postaural hearing aid.

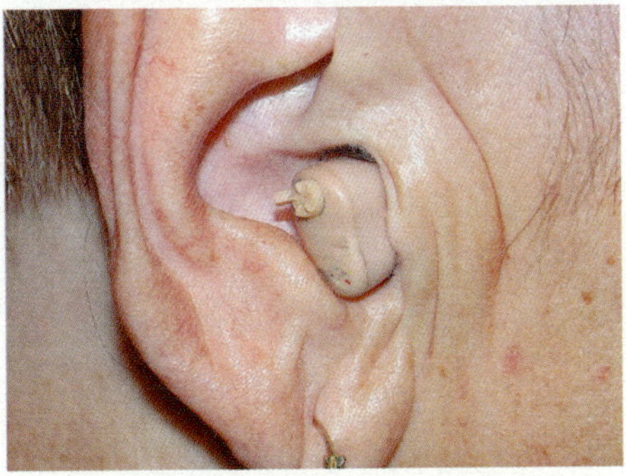

图 56　耳内式助听器
An 'in the ear' hearing aid.

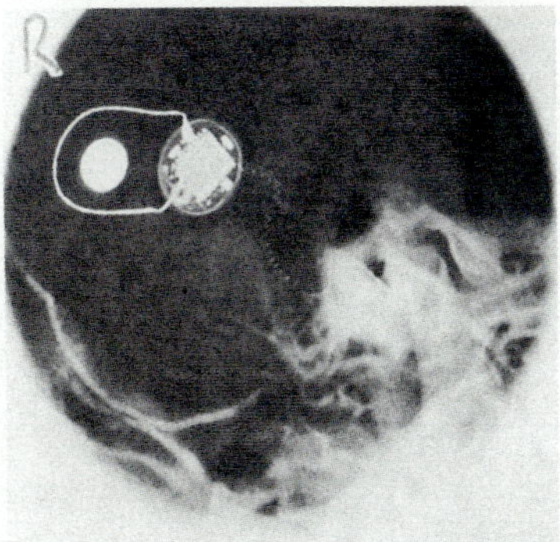

图 57　X 线平片显示植入后的电子耳蜗
X-ray showing cochlear implant in situ.

17 鼻的临床检查

鼻塞、流涕、鼻出血或面部疼痛是鼻腔或鼻窦疾病的常见症状。临床检查应先从视诊开始。观察患者的呼吸情况，患者是强制性张口呼吸吗？观察外鼻有无畸形，检查鼻腔通气情况。儿童可用铬压舌板放在鼻孔下方，同时让患儿呼吸（图58）。如果在压舌板上有一层薄雾，表示鼻腔通气；成人可用拇指每次阻塞一个鼻孔，观察鼻腔通气情况，注意不要侧压以免同时将双侧鼻孔阻塞。

然后再用前鼻镜检查双侧鼻腔。在评估鼻腔外侧壁情况的同时，也要评估鼻中隔前部的情况（图59），同时还应注意鼻腔黏膜有无炎症。前鼻镜下三个鼻甲只能看到中鼻甲和下鼻甲。

最后检查鼻咽部，压舌板压舌前2/3，用间接鼻咽镜检查鼻咽部和咽鼓管开口。检查有困难者，可用纤维内镜检查。

如果有可疑病变，亦应对耳、喉、颈进行相应检查。

Clinical examination of the nose

Nasal obstruction, rhinorrhoea, epistaxis or facial pain may indicate intranasal or paranasal sinus disease. Clinical assessment begins with observation. Is the patient an obligatory mouth breather? Look for an obvious external nasal deformity. The nasal airway is then assessed. In children, this is undertaken using a chrome tongue depressor held just below the nose whilst the child breathes (Fig. 58). Misting of the chrome indicates a patent airway. In adults the examiner's thumb is used to close one airway at a time, being careful not to apply any lateral pressure that could occlude both sides simultaneously.

The two nasal cavities are then examined in turn using a Thudicums nasal speculum. The anterior nasal septum is assessed along with evaluation of the lateral nasal walls (Fig. 59). Only the inferior and middle turbinates can be seen by anterior rhinoscopy. The nasal mucosa is also evaluated for evidence of rhinitis.

Finally, the nasopharynx is examined. A tongue depressor is used to allow mirror examination of the nasopharynx and Eustachian tube orifices. Alternatively, fibreoptic endoscopy can be employed.

Depending on the suspected pathology, the ears, larynx and neck should also be assessed.

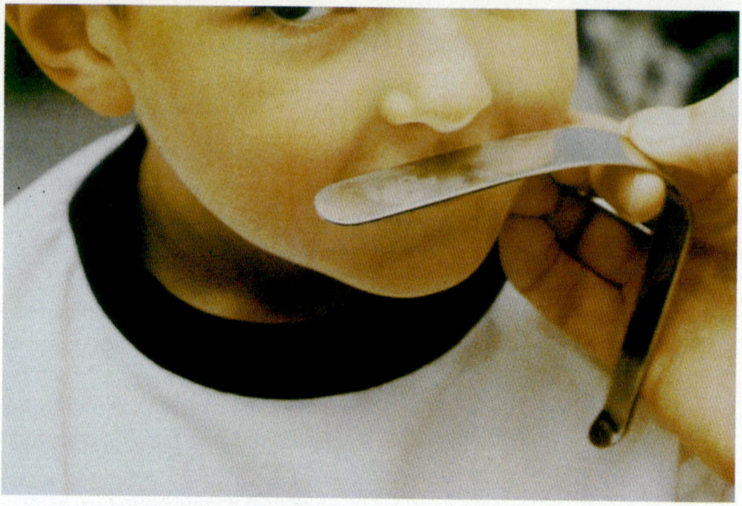

图 58　儿童鼻通气情况的检查
Assessing the child's nasal airway.

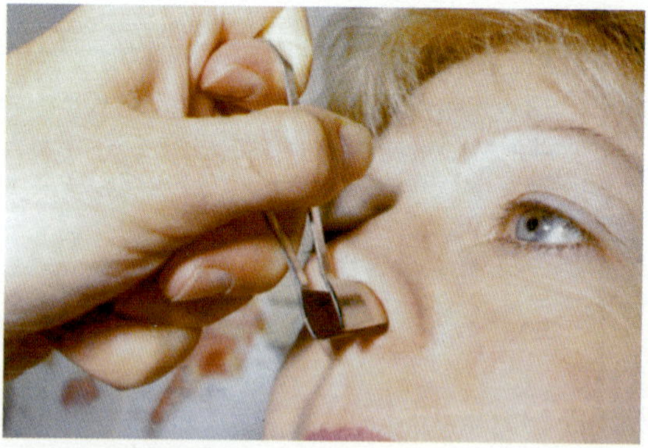

图 59　鼻腔检查
Examining the nasal cavities.

肥大性酒渣鼻

临床特征 以鼻尖为中心红色结节状皮赘，常伴红斑、痤疮（图60）。老年人多见。

治疗 如果影响外观，需切除或手术整形。

寻常狼疮

病因 可能为用手挖鼻引起的结核分支杆菌的种植。

临床特征 鼻或面部皮肤红色/褐色斑或小结。病期长者可发生软骨鼻中隔穿孔（图61）、瘢痕形成。

治疗 抗结核菌化学治疗。

冻疮样狼疮

临床特征 20%类肉瘤病的患者，可发生与结节性红斑不同的皮损。冻疮样狼疮（图62）较常见，常与骨囊肿和胸部疾病有关。

治疗 积极治疗基础疾病。

恶性肿瘤

临床特征 基底细胞癌或鳞状细胞癌（图63）常表现为疣状或溃疡性皮损。极少发生淋巴结转移。黑色素瘤更少见。

治疗 尽可能完全切除送活组织检查，肿瘤较大但未侵及骨壁者可行放射治疗。

18 Diseases of the external nose

Rhinophyma

Clinical features Red nodular masses centred around the nasal tip in association with acne rosacea (Fig. 60), usually seen in elderly men.

Management If unsightly, treat by dermabrasion or surgical shaving.

Lupus vulgaris

Aetiology Inoculation of the bacterium *Mycobacterium tuberculosis*, possibly through nose picking.

Clinical features Red/brown patches or nodules on the nasal or facial skin. Perforation of the cartilaginous nasal septum can occur, with scarring in long-standing cases (Fig. 61).

Management Treatment is by antituberculous chemotherapy.

Lupus pernio

Clinical features Skin lesions other than erythema nodosum occur in 20% of patients with sarcoidosis. Lupus pernio (Fig. 62) is common and is frequently associated with bone cysts and chest disease.

Management Treat the underlying disease.

Malignant tumours

Clinical features Basal or squamous cell carcinomas (Fig. 63) present as warty or ulcerating lesions, rarely with lymphadenopathy. Melanomas are more rare.

Management Excision biopsy when possible; radiotherapy for larger tumours not involving bone.

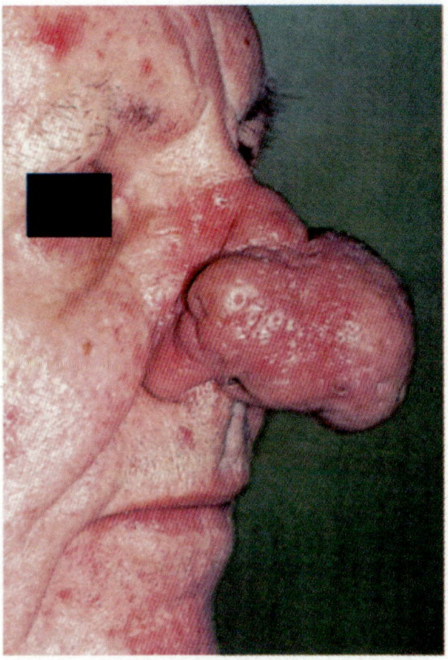

图 60　肥大性酒渣鼻
Rhinophyma.

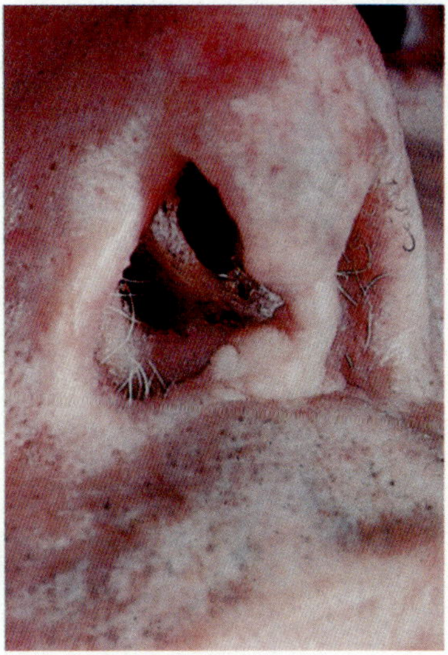

图 61　寻常狼疮
Lupus vulgaris.

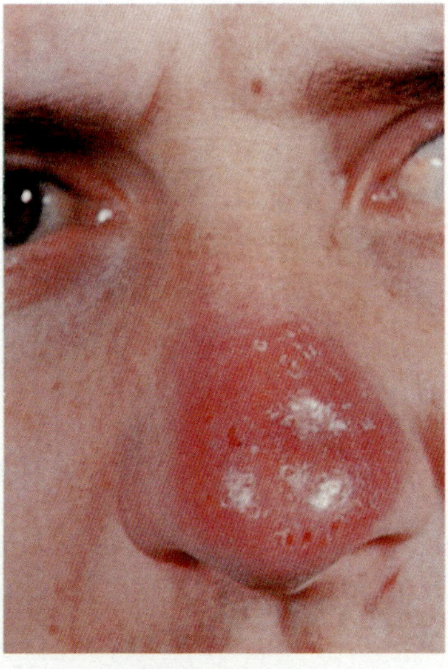

图 62　冻疮样狼疮
Lupus pernio.

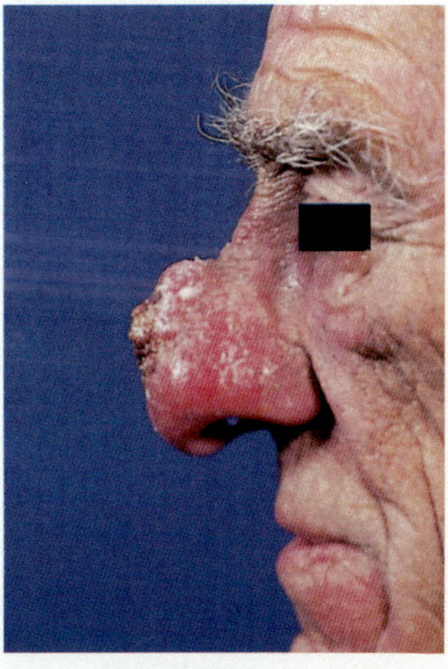

图 63　鳞状细胞癌
Squamous carcinoma.

19 鼻出血

病因

大多数鼻出血是原发性的，也有少数患者是因特定疾病引起的。

局部因素：鼻外伤、鼻和鼻窦肿瘤以及鼻中隔穿孔。

全身因素：包括全身有出血倾向的患者，如白血病、抗凝治疗、血小板减少症和系统性血管异常；在遗传性出血性毛细血管扩张症（又称Rendu-Osler-Weber综合征，图 64）的患者中，鼻出血是最突出的临床特征，通常由鼻中隔上异常的血管引起。高血压病虽然不是鼻出血的原因，但常与鼻出血的严重程度有关。

临床特征

大多数鼻出血来自鼻中隔，多见于黎氏区（Little's area）。黎氏区恰位于鼻中隔皮肤与黏膜交界处的后方，该区的血管丰富，各分支相互吻合形成血管网(Kiesselbach's plexus，图 65)。鼻出血也可发生在鼻腔的后上部分，老年人多见。鼻出血可经前鼻孔流出，也可向后流经鼻咽部吐出或咽下。大量失血的患者，可发生低血压和心动过速。

Epistaxis 19

Aetiology

Most cases of epistaxis are idiopathic, although bleeding can also result from a number of specific conditions.

Local conditions include nasal trauma, nasal and paranasal sinus tumours and nasal septal perforations.

General conditions include systemic bleeding diatheses such as leukaemia, anticoagulant therapy and thrombocytopenia, and systemic vascular disorders. In hereditary haemorrhagic telangiectasia (Rendu-Osler-Weber syndrome, Fig. 64), epistaxis is a prominent feature and usually arises from abnormal vessels on the nasal septum.

Systemic hypertension, although not a cause of epistaxis, is often associated with an increased severity of bleeding.

Clinical features

In most cases of epistaxis bleeding originates from the nasal septum, particularly Little's area just behind the mucocutaneous junction where there is a rich anastomosis of vessels (Kiesselbach's plexus, Fig. 65). Bleeding from a postero-superior site in the nasal cavity can occur, especially in the elderly. Haemorrhage can present via the anterior nares or pass backwards via the nasopharynx where it is spat out or swallowed. In severe cases with profuse blood loss, hypotension and tachycardia may occur.

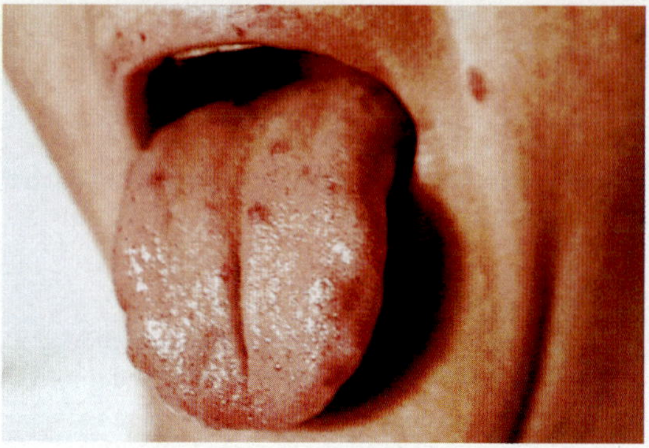

图 64　Rendu-Osler-Weber 综合征
Rendu-Osler-Weber syndrome.

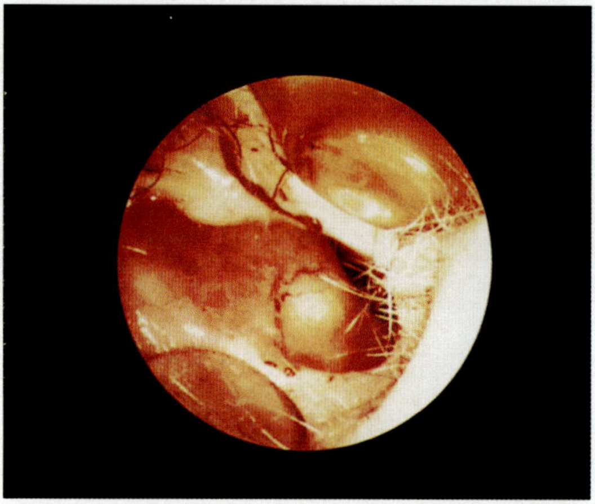

图 65　鼻内镜下显示黎氏区的血管网
Endoscopic view of prominent blood vessels in Little's area.

治疗

1. 一般处理：患者坐位前倾，用手挤压双侧鼻翼压迫黎氏区，阻止出血。血要尽量吐出，不要咽下（图66）。
2. 烧灼法：如果能看到出血点，可在局麻下用化学药物烧灼或电凝，但在急性期很难将其凝固。
3. 鼻腔填塞：如果指压不能控制出血，应用浸有防腐软膏（如铋、碘仿和石蜡，即BIPP）的纱条填塞或用气囊充填（图67）。需要填塞的患者亦需住院治疗。
4. 动脉结扎或栓塞：严重病例可行动脉结扎。目前最常用的方法是鼻内镜下蝶腭动脉结扎或电凝。其他方法还有颈外动脉结扎术（图68）和经内眦筛前动脉结扎术。出血严重者也可由影像学医师行血管造影动脉栓塞术。
5. 全身治疗：如出血较多，发生低血压或心动过速，应静脉输血或血浆代用品补充血容量。

Management

Initial measures to stop bleeding consist of exerting pressure on Little's area by pinching the nose, with the patient leaning forward and spitting any blood into a bowl (Fig. 66). If a bleeding vessel is seen, it may be coagulated with chemical or electric cautery following topical application of local anaesthetic, but this is rarely successful in the acute stage. Epistaxis not responding to pressure necessitates nasal packing either with gauze impregnated with an antiseptic such as bismuth, iodoform and paraffin paste (BIPP) (Fig. 67) or with nasal balloons. Patients requiring nasal packing also require hospitalization.

In severe cases arterial ligation may be required. Endoscopic ligation or diathermy of the sphenopalatine artery in the nasal cavity is the commonest method. Other available arteries are the external carotid via the neck (Fig. 68) and the anterior ethmoidal via an inner canthal incision.

An alternative to arterial ligation in severe cases is arterial embolization performed with angiographic control by a radiologist. Intravenous resuscitation with blood or plasma substitute is necessary in cases where hypotension and tachycardia are present.

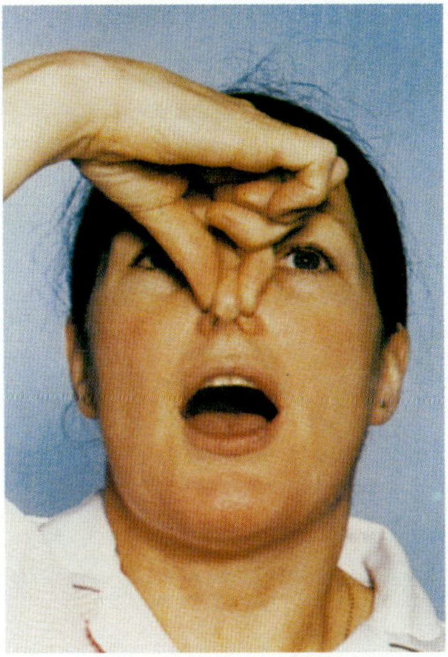

图 66 鼻出血时的体位与指压法
Pressure and posture during epistaxis.

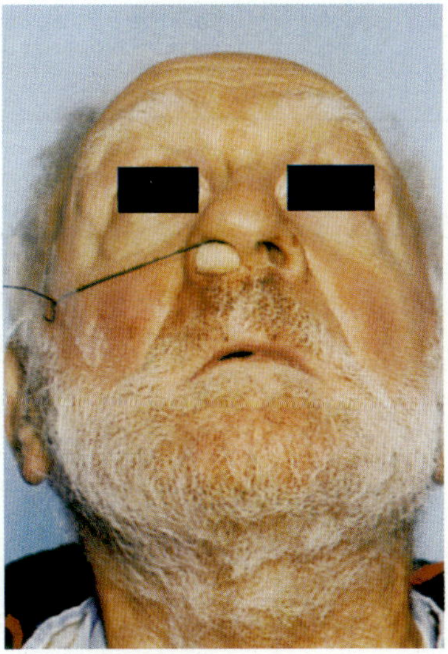

图 67 鼻腔填塞
Nasal packing.

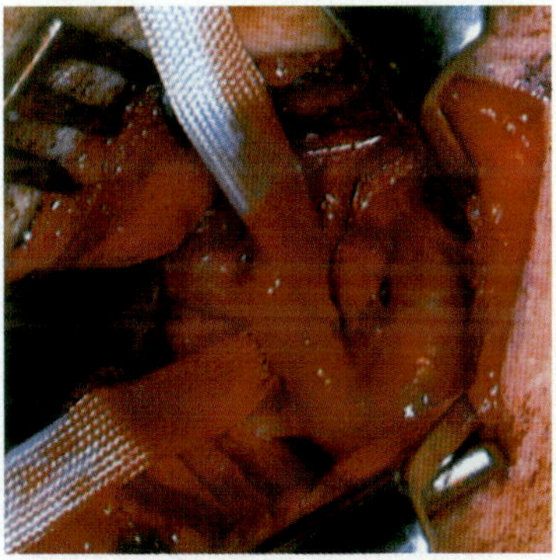

图 68 结扎前显露的颈外动脉
External carotid artery just prior to ligation.

鼻中隔疾病

鼻中隔偏曲

病因 外伤或出生时产伤所致的鼻中隔不对称性发育。

临床特征 多为单侧鼻堵（图69），少数表现为鼻出血。鼻中隔偏曲的对侧中鼻甲和下鼻甲常有代偿性肥厚。

治疗 如果症状与鼻中隔偏曲有关，应矫正鼻中隔，方法有鼻中隔成形术和鼻中隔黏膜下切除术。

鼻中隔血肿

鼻中隔血肿是指鼻中隔黏膜软骨膜下和后方黏膜骨膜下的积血。

病因 多因鼻外伤引起，如事故或鼻中隔手术造成的医源性血肿。因出血性疾病引起的自发性血肿在临床上较为少见。

临床特征 鼻堵。鼻腔检查可见鼻中隔膨隆变宽（图70）。

治疗 急性期应切开引流，但若超过48小时，血肿机化，血块清除较困难。全身应用抗生素预防继发感染。

Diseases of the nasal septum

Deviated nasal septum

Aetiology

This occurs following previous nasal trauma or results from asymmetric septal development possibly following birth trauma.

Clinical features

Presents as unilateral nasal obstruction (Fig. 69) and less commonly epistaxis. The inferior and middle turbinates on the side opposite the septal deflection often undergo compensatory hypertrophy.

Management

If symptoms warrant, the septum can be positioned in the midline as in the operations of septoplasty and submucosal resection.

Septal haematoma

A collection of blood beneath the mucoperichondrium and posteriorly the mucoperiosteum of the nasal septum.

Aetiology

Usually complicates nasal trauma, either accidental or iatrogenic following septal surgery. Rarely a spontaneous haematoma can occur in a bleeding diathesis.

Clinical features

Presents as nasal obstruction with widening of the septum on inspection (Fig. 70).

Management

In the acute stage, treat by incision and drainage; however, after 48h, organization of haematoma occurs and evacuation of the clot is difficult. Antibiotics are given to prevent secondary infection.

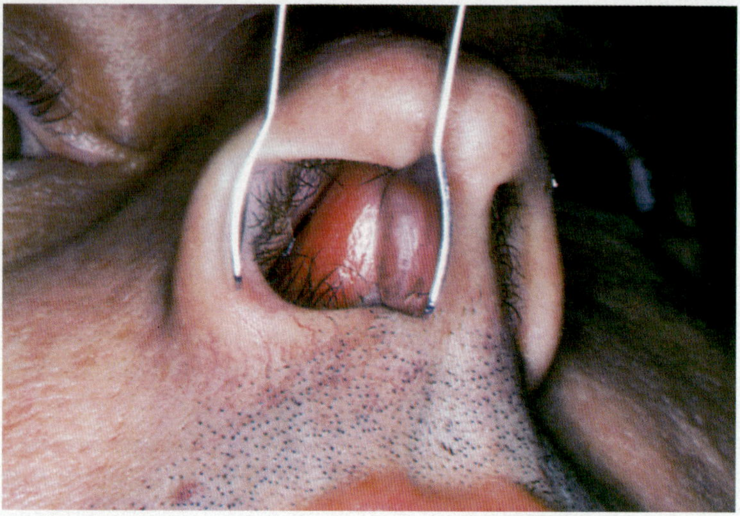

图 69　鼻中隔偏曲
Deviated nasal septum.

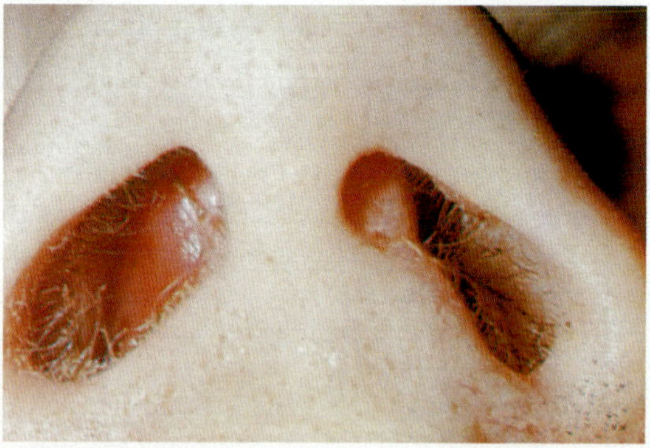

图 70　鼻中隔血肿
Septal haematoma.

鼻中隔脓肿

病因 大多由鼻中隔血肿继发感染而引起。

临床特征 鼻中隔血肿后出现发热、鼻部隆突、重度疼痛。鼻中隔血肿和脓肿可导致软骨坏死，形成鞍鼻畸形（图 71）。

治疗 切开引流，适当应用抗生素治疗。

鼻中隔穿孔

病因 *外伤*：鼻中隔手术后，挖鼻，鼻吸可卡因，异物和鼻息肉的压迫。

感染：梅毒和结核感染。

慢性炎症：Wegener肉芽肿是伴有病灶性肺和肾损害的非新生物性上呼吸道肉芽肿。（致死性）中线肉芽肿一般认为是发生于面中线的非典型性淋巴瘤。

临床特征 一般无明显症状，部分患者有鼻内结痂和鼻出血（图 72）。

治疗 去除干痂，鼻腔冲洗，根据全身情况治疗基础疾病。

Septal abscess

Aetiology

Septal abscesses usually result from secondary infection of a septal haematoma.

Clinical features

Manifests by the development of severe pain, nasal swelling and pyrexia following a septal haematoma. Cartilage necrosis often complicates septal haematoma and abscess with the production of a saddle-nose deformity (Fig. 71).

Management

Treatment is by incision and drainage with appropriate antibiotic therapy.

Septal perforation

Aetiology

Traumatic: after septal surgery, nose picking, cocaine sniffing and pressure from foreign bodies and nasal polyps.

Infective: due to syphilis and tuberculosis.

Chronic inflammatory. Wegener's granulomatosis is a non-neoplastic upper airways granuloma associated with focal lung and kidney lesions. (Lethal) midline granuloma is thought to be an atypical lymphoma occurring in the midline of the face.

Clinical features

Asymptomatic, or nasal crusting and epistaxis are characteristic of septal perforation (Fig. 72).

Management

Treatment is by removal of crusts, nasal douches and treatment of underlying systemic conditions.

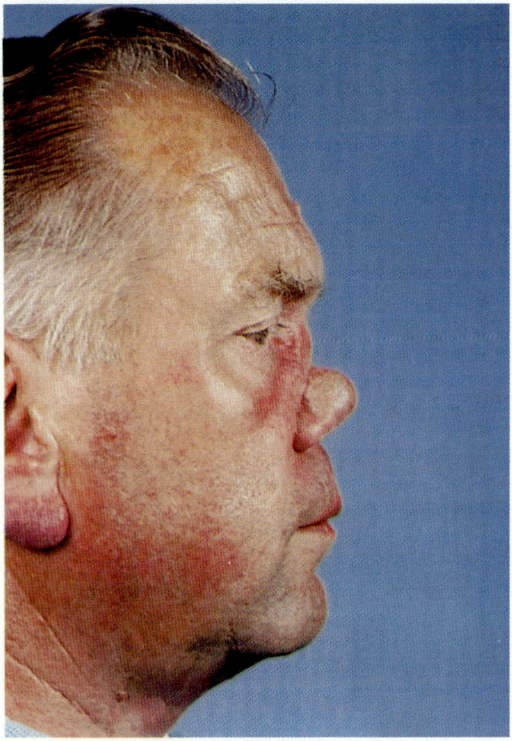

图 71 鼻中隔脓肿后鞍鼻畸形
Saddle-nose deformity following septal abscess.

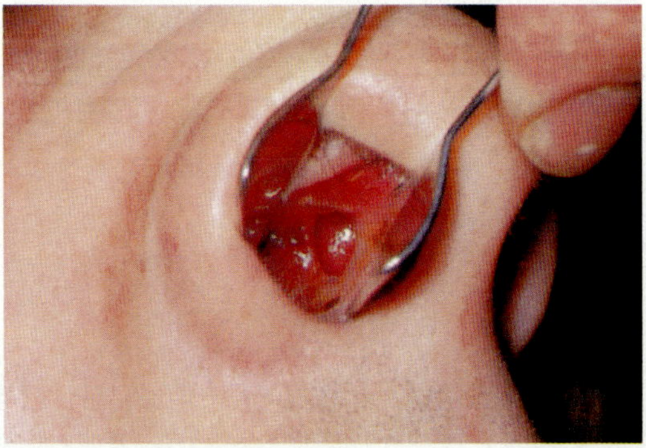

图 72 鼻中隔穿孔
Septal perforation.

21 非感染性鼻炎

变应性鼻炎

病因 变应性鼻炎是指对某些吸入性或食入性变应原反应过于敏感，而引起的鼻黏膜水肿和渗出。变应性鼻炎可表现为季节性（如花粉），也可为常年性（如屋尘）。过敏反应可通过皮肤试验来确定（图 73）。

临床特征 鼻堵、打喷嚏、流清涕、鼻腔检查鼻黏膜肿胀（图 74）。

治疗 类固醇激素鼻喷剂，口服抗组胺药，避免接触过敏原。

非变应性鼻炎

临床特征 慢性鼻堵和流涕而无明确的过敏原。

治疗 如果应用抗组胺药或鼻内类固醇激素喷雾治疗效果不满意，鼻堵症状可通过下鼻甲部分切除术或热凝治疗改善。如果长期应用拟交感神经血管收缩药，由于其反跳作用，可导致鼻黏膜的慢性充血，形成药物性鼻炎。

萎缩性鼻炎

病因 病因不明。多发生在发展中国家。也可发生于过多切除下鼻甲的手术或鼻腔放疗后。

临床特征 鼻内结痂、失嗅和臭鼻症。虽然鼻腔宽大，但患者常有鼻堵的感觉。

治疗 清除干痂和鼻腔冲洗。

Non-infective rhinitis

Allergic rhinitis

Aetiology — Hypersensitivity to inhaled or ingested allergens causes nasal mucosal oedema and exudation. Allergy may be seasonal (e. g. pollens) or perennial (e.g. house dust). Allergies may be demonstrated by skin tests (Fig. 73).

Clinical features — Presents as nasal obstruction, sneezing and rhinorrhoea with mucosal oedema on examination (Fig. 74).

Management — Treat with steroid nasal spray and oral antihistamines. Avoid any known allergens.

Non-allergic rhinitis

Clinical features — Presents as chronic nasal obstruction and rhinorrhoea with no demonstrable allergy.

Management — If medical treatment in the form of antihistamines or steroid sprays fails to produce relief, nasal obstruction may be helped by surgical reduction or diathermy of the inferior turbinates. Long term use of sympathomimetic vasoconstrictor nasal sprays can result in chronic nasal congestion as a rebound effect: rhinitis medicamentosa.

Atrophic rhinitis

Aetiology — A disease of unknown aetiology, occurring mainly in developing countries. It can occur following radical turbinectomy operations or radiotherapy to the nasal cavity.

Clinical features — Nasal crusting, anosmia and fetor are present. Paradoxically, although the nasal cavity is widely patent, the sensation of nasal obstruction is common.

Management — Treatment is by removal of crusts and nasal douches.

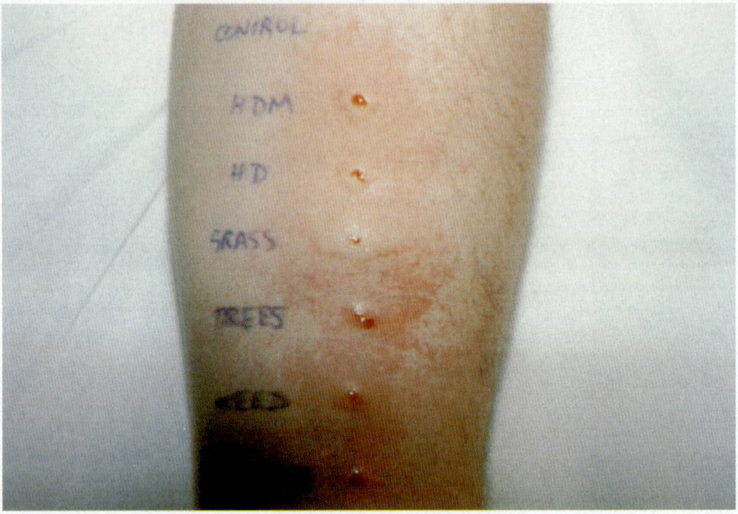

图 73　变应性鼻炎，皮肤试验阳性
Positive skin tests in allergic rhinitis.

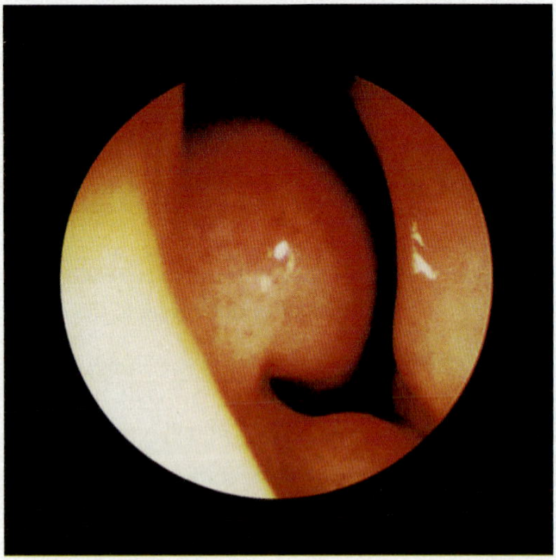

图 74　下鼻甲肥大
Inferior turbinate hypertrophy.

22 鼻息肉

病因

鼻息肉是鼻腔和鼻窦黏膜水肿脱垂形成的带蒂的息肉。本病病因不清，可能与慢性鼻窦感染和鼻黏膜的变态反应有关。大多数的息肉来自筛窦，少数来自上颌窦口。

鼻息肉还与哮喘和阿司匹林耐受不良有关（阿司匹林三联征）。儿童鼻息肉可能是囊性纤维性变的表现。

临床特征

渐进性鼻堵、流涕。

鼻腔检查可见灰白色、光滑肿物，可充满鼻腔（图75）。大多数患者是双侧的，单侧鼻息肉需活检排除肿瘤。上颌窦后鼻孔息肉来自上颌窦经其自然口向后坠入后鼻孔，通过后鼻镜（图76）可以看到，亦可辅以头颅X线侧位片检查。

治疗

*药物治疗：*正确使用局部类固醇激素喷雾或滴剂可使鼻息肉明显缩小。

*手术治疗：*单纯鼻息肉摘除术后常易复发（图77），目前多主张鼻内镜下筛窦切除术，经筛窦彻底切除息肉。

22 Simple nasal polyps

Aetiology

Simple nasal polyps are pedunculated areas of oedematous mucosa occurring in the nasal cavity and paranasal sinuses. Their aetiology is unknown although chronic sinus infection and mucosal allergy have been suggested. Most polyps arise from the ethmoid sinuses with the maxillary antrum being a less common source.

Nasal polyps can be associated with asthma and aspirin sensitivity (aspirin triad). In children, nasal polyps may be a manifestation of cystic fibrosis.

Clinical features

Presents as progressive nasal obstruction and rhinorrhoea. On inspection of the nasal cavity, polyps are seen as pale grey, smooth swellings, which can fill the nasal cavity (Fig. 75). Most cases are bilateral but in unilateral cases a neoplasm must be excluded by biopsy. An antrochoanal polyp passes from the maxillary sinus via its ostium posteriorly into the nasal cavity to occupy the posterior choana where it can be seen on posterior rhinoscopy (Fig. 76) and its presence confirmed by lateral radiography.

Management

Medical treatment: topical steroid drops or spray administered correctly can cause considerable diminution in polyp size.

Surgical treatment: intranasal polypectomy (Fig. 77) may have to be repeated as recurrence after polyp removal is common. Many surgeons use endoscopic ethmoidectomy techniques to remove polyps from the ethmoid sinuses.

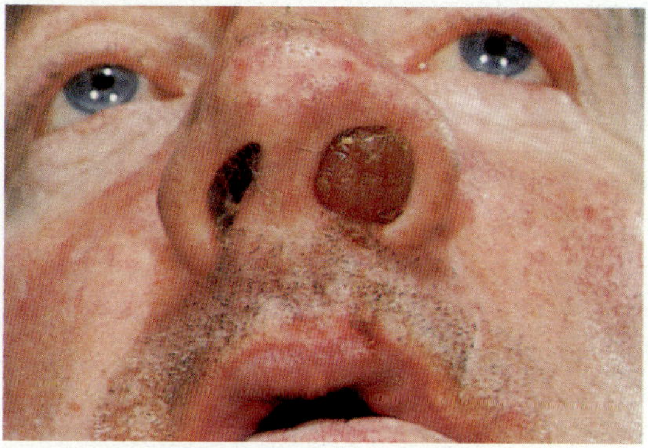

图 75 单发性鼻息肉
Simple nasal polyps.

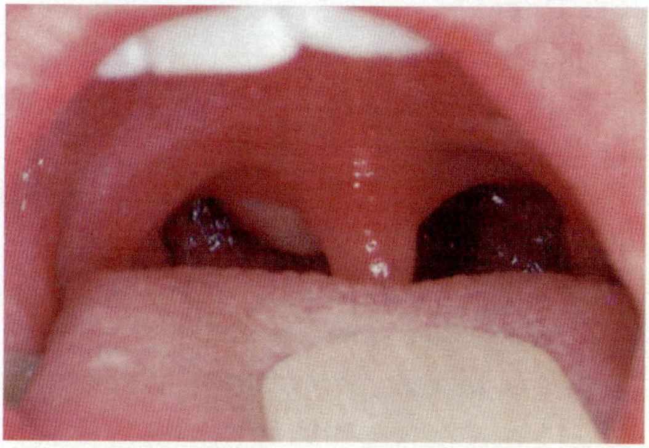

图 76 软腭后方的上颌窦 - 后鼻孔息肉
Antrochoanal polyp behind soft palate.

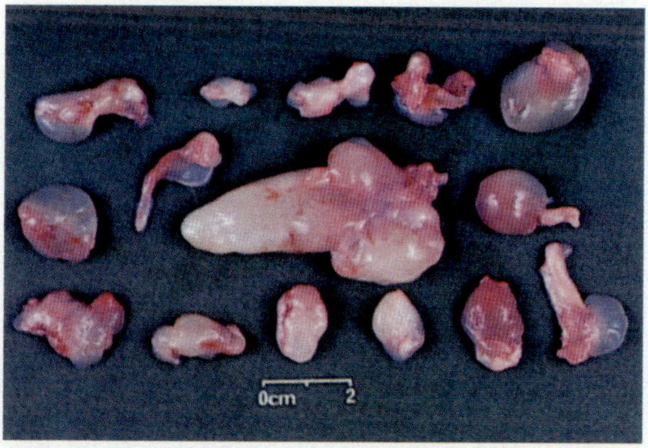

图 77 同一个患者的鼻息肉标本
Operative specimens from one patient.

23 急性鼻窦炎

病因

鼻腔鼻窦的病理改变或解剖异常可影响鼻窦的通气引流，从而导致鼻窦分泌物的潴留和急性感染。上呼吸道感染是最常见的诱因，上列牙齿的根尖感染可引起急性上颌窦炎。病原菌多为肺炎双球菌、溶血性链球菌或流感嗜血杆菌。

并发症

急性鼻窦炎治疗不及时最易迁延形成慢性鼻窦炎。其他少见的并发症有眶蜂窝织炎、海绵窦血栓或颅内脓肿形成（图 78）。

上颌窦炎

临床特征

是最常见的类型，多伴有面痛或牙痛，也可引起反射性耳痛。常见的症状是鼻堵和脓涕；有时局部触痛可能是惟一的阳性体征。枕颏位 X 线片显示一侧或双侧鼻窦内液平（图 79），但目前 X 线片已逐渐被 CT 所取代（图 80）。

治疗

抗生素治疗；
局部鼻内减充血剂；
如果经抗生素治疗炎症仍未消退，可经下鼻道行上颌窦穿刺冲洗（图 81）。但随着鼻内镜手术的普遍开展，这种治疗方法的应用逐渐减少。

Acute sinusitis

Aetiology

Stasis and acute infection of sinus secretions may result from any pathological or anatomical abnormality obstructing free sinus drainage. The common cold is the most frequent cause. Acute maxillary sinusitis can also result from apical infection of an upper tooth root. The causative organism is usually *Pneumococcus*, *Streptococcus viridans* or *Haemophilus influenzae*.

Complications

Left untreated, acute sinusitis can rarely lead to orbital cellulitis, cavernous sinus thrombosis or intracranial abscess formation (Fig. 78). Chronic sinusitis is a far more common sequela.

Maxillary sinusitis

Clinical features

Most common type overall. Facial or dental pain may occur, as may referred otalgia. Nasal obstruction and purulent rhinorrhoea are also frequent. Local tenderness may be the only physical sign. An occipitomental X-ray usually shows a fluid level on one or both sides (Fig. 79), but this investigation is increasingly being replaced by CT scanning (Fig. 80).

Management

Treat with antibiotics and topical nasal decongestants. An antral washout (Fig. 81) through the inferior meatus may be necessary if resolution with antibiotics does not occur, but this form of treatment is decreasing in popularity with the advent of endoscopic management of sinusitis.

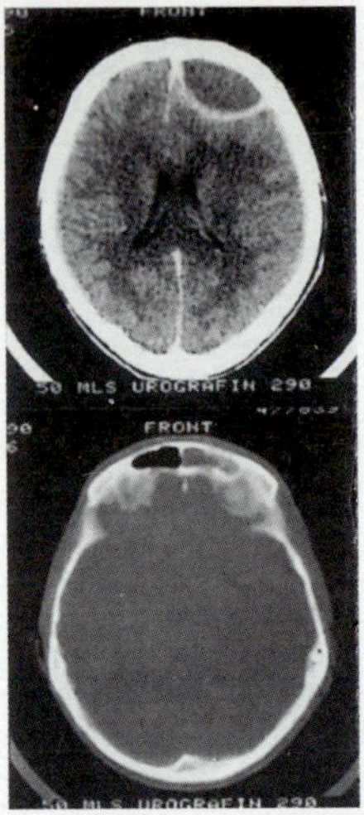

图 78　前颅窝硬脑膜外脓肿（上图）继发于额窦炎（下图）
Anterior fossa extradural abscess (upper scan) secondary to frontal sinusitis (lower scan).

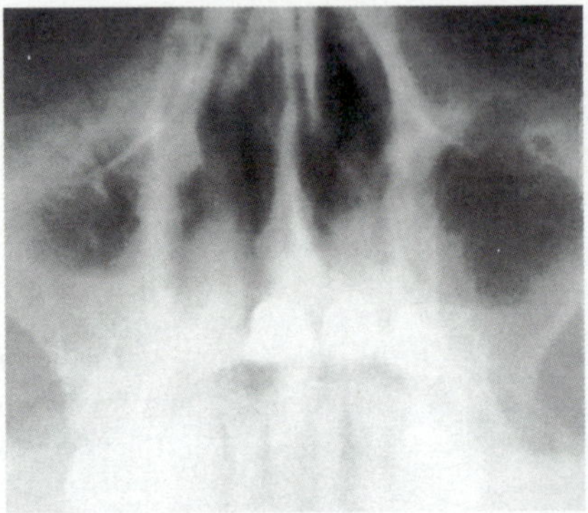

图 79　双侧上颌窦液平
Bilateral antral fluid levels.

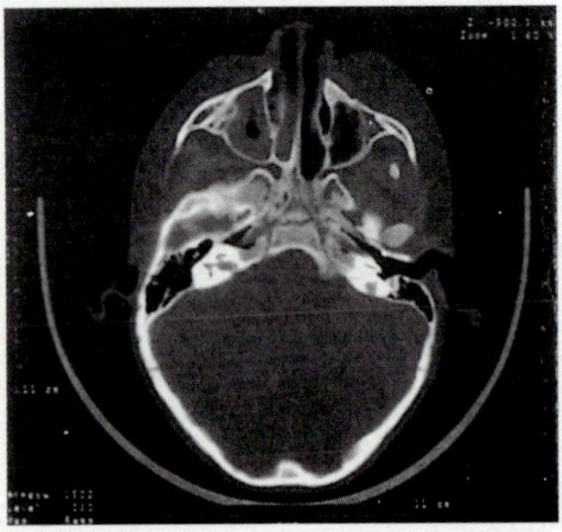

图 80　CT 显示上颌窦炎
CT scan of maxillary sinusitis.

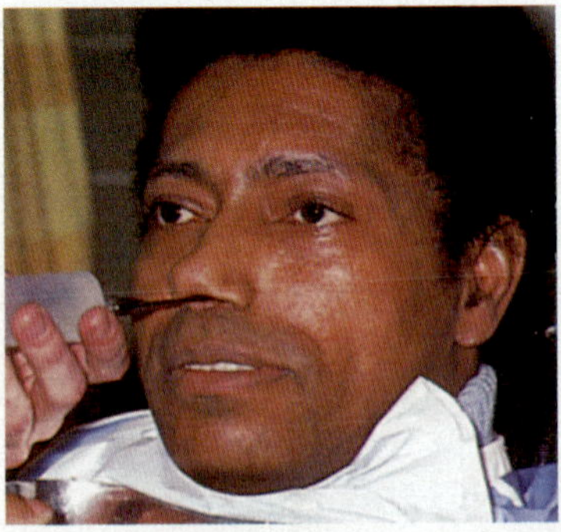

图 81　上颌窦穿刺冲洗
Antral washout.

筛窦炎

发病率 最常见于上颌窦发育不良的儿童。

临床特征 上呼吸道感染后出现持续性头痛和眶蜂窝织炎（图82），如不及时治疗可导致眶脓肿和失明。

治疗 一般需住院治疗，应用抗生素。如果合并上颌窦感染可行上颌窦穿刺冲洗。极少数患者需行鼻外筛窦切除术。如果疑有眶脓肿，应进行 CT 扫描检查。

额窦炎

是急性鼻窦炎中最严重的一种类型。由于鼻额管较长，易被肿胀的黏膜阻塞。

临床特征 上呼吸道感染后出现前额部疼痛。局部触痛是常见的体征，也可能是惟一的阳性体征。鼻窦CT扫描可显示一侧或双侧额窦内液平或整个窦腔模糊浑浊。

治疗 全身应用抗生素治疗，如果症状不缓解，可采取额窦钻孔插管引流术（图 83）。

蝶窦炎

临床特征 较少见，表现为头颅深部中央、眶后或头顶疼痛。头颅侧位片或 CT 扫描（图 84）可帮助诊断。如果抗生素治疗不缓解，应行鼻窦引流术。

Ethmoiditis

Incidence

Most common in young children who have poorly developed maxillary sinuses.

Clinical features

Usually presents as persistent headache and orbital cellulitis (Fig. 82) following a cold. Untreated, an orbital abscess and blindness may occur.

Management

Treatment requires hospital admission. Antibiotics are given and the maxillary sinuses washed out if also infected. Rarely, an external ethmoidectomy may be necessary. A CT scan should be performed if there is any question of an orbital abscess.

Frontal sinusitis

Potentially the most serious acute sinusitis. The long course of the frontonasal duct makes it particularly prone to obstruction by mucosal oedema.

Clinical features

Presents as frontal headache after an upper respiratory tract infection. Local tenderness is common, but may be the only sign. A sinus CT scan usually shows a fluid level or complete opacification in one or both sinuses.

Management

Treatment is with antibiotics, but sinus trephine and insertion of drainage tubes (Fig. 83) is undertaken if rapid resolution does not occur.

Sphenoiditis

Clinical features

This rare form of sinusitis may present as a deep central, retro-orbital or vertex headache. Diagnosis is confirmed by a lateral X-ray or CT scan (Fig. 84). Sinus drainage may be necessary if there is not a quick response to antibiotic therapy.

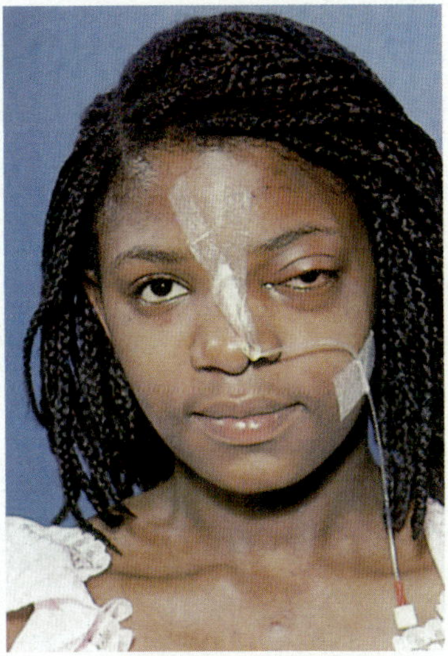

图 82　急性筛窦炎合并眶蜂窝织炎
Acute ethmoiditis with orbital cellulitis.

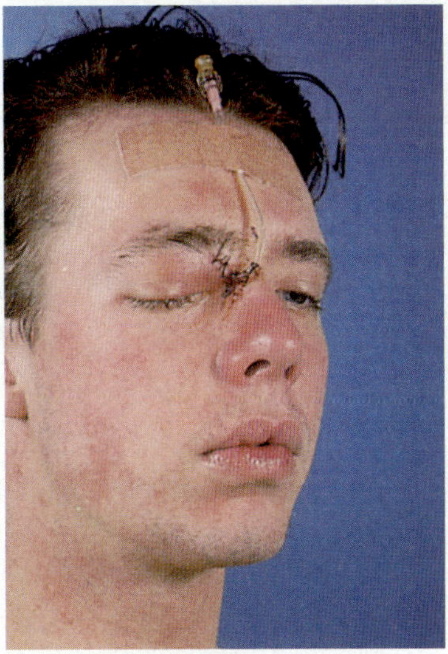

图 83　急性额窦炎手术引流
Surgical drainage of acute frontal sinusitis.

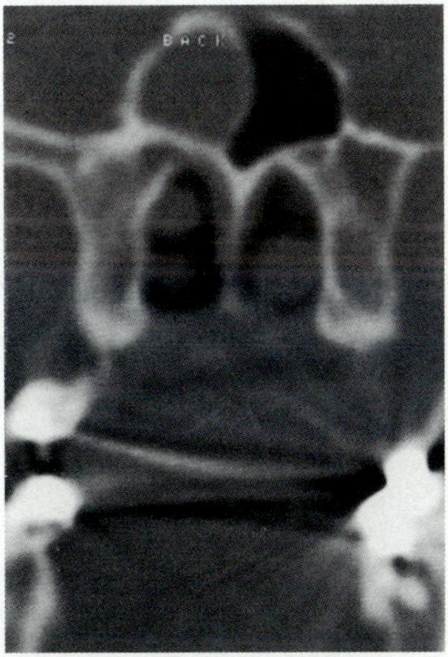

图 84　CT 显示蝶窦黏液囊肿
Sphenoid sinus mucocele on CT scan.

慢性鼻窦炎

额窦炎

临床特征

持续的前额痛。如果发生黏液囊肿，可引起单侧眼球突出（图 85）。黏液囊肿继发感染即形成脓囊肿。鼻窦X线片显示不透光影，边界常模糊不清。CT扫描显示鼻窦软组织影（图 86）。

治疗

手术治疗的目的是重建额窦的通气引流。进入与额窦交通的额隐窝区域，可通过鼻内镜手术，也可经鼻外径路进入。而额窦根治性手术如骨壁成形额窦填塞术目前已很少应用。

上颌窦炎

病因

除因鼻中隔偏曲、单侧鼻息肉或上颌骨外伤引起单侧上颌窦炎外，一般多为双侧病变。有时还与既往的牙齿治疗史有关。

临床特征

常有慢性面部疼痛或上列牙痛。其他临床表现有：脓涕倒流、慢性喉炎或中耳炎。鼻腔检查常无异常所见，但鼻窦 X 线检查可显示鼻窦内病变，如黏膜增厚、持续性液平或窦腔浑浊。

治疗

经鼻行鼻窦造口术，改善窦口的通气引流。目前多在内镜下经中鼻道行上颌窦窦口扩大术。严重病例可通过柯 - 陆氏手术去除鼻窦的病变黏膜（图 87）。

Chronic sinusitis

Frontal sinusitis

Clinical features

Presents as a persistent frontal headache or, if a mucocele develops, a unilateral proptosis (Fig. 85). A pyocele may result from secondary infection of a mucocele. X-rays show an opaque sinus, often with hazy, indistinct edges. A CT scan will show a soft tissue mass filling the sinus (Fig. 86).

Management

Surgical treatment is aimed at re-establishing aeration of the frontal sinus. The area of the frontal recess leading into the frontal sinus can be approached either endoscopically through the nasal cavity or via an external incision. Obliteration of the frontal sinus via an osteoplastic flap approach is a radical proceduce very rarely required.

Maxillary sinusitis

Aetiology

Disease is commonly bilateral unless there is an underlying septal deviation, unilateral polyp or history of maxillary trauma. A past history of dental treatment may be relevant.

Clinical features

Usually presents with chronic facial pain or upper jaw toothache. Other presentations include a purulent postnasal drip, chronic laryngitis or otitis media. Examination is often normal but paranasal sinus X-rays usually demonstrate antral disease, in the form of mucosal thickening, a persistent fluid level or total opacification.

Management

Treatment involves the creation of intranasal antrostomies to ventilate and drain the antra. Antrostomies are now normally performed endoscopically through the middle meatus. In severe cases a Caldwell-Luc approach can be used to remove diseased antral mucosa (Fig. 87).

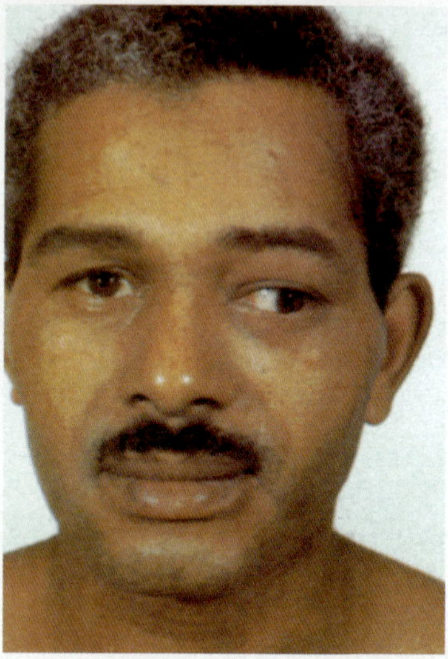

图 85　黏液囊肿引起的单侧眼球突出
Unilateral proptosis due to a mucocele.

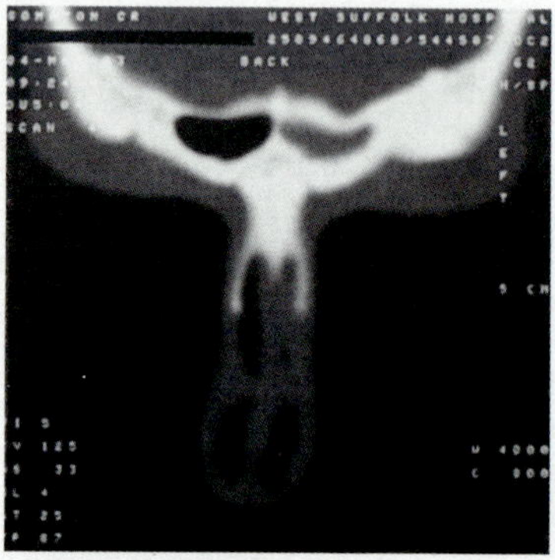

图 86　单侧慢性额窦炎
Unilateral chronic frontal sinusitis.

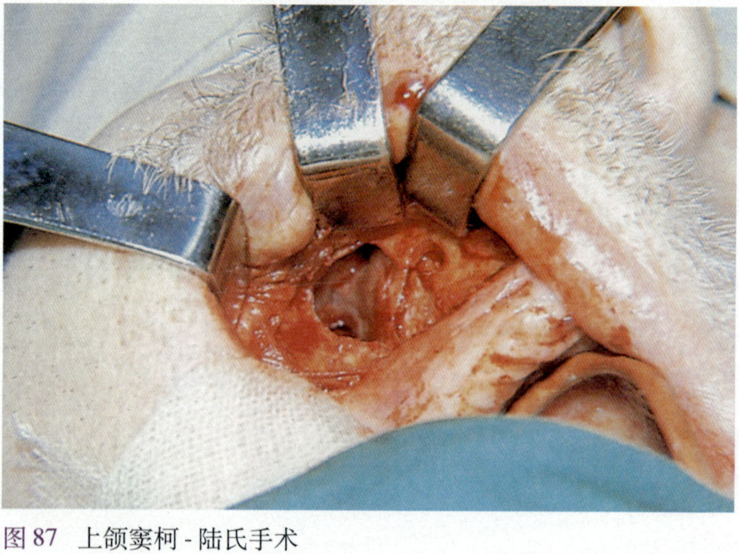

图 87　上颌窦柯 - 陆氏手术
Caldwell-Luc approach to the maxillary antrum.

功能性鼻窦内镜手术

随着内镜技术和高质量放射学的普遍应用，人们对以往慢性鼻窦炎的多种治疗方法进行重新评估。大多数的鼻窦感染是鼻源性的，即从鼻腔蔓延至鼻窦。额窦和上颌窦是通过邻近中鼻甲、前组筛窦的狭窄裂隙进行通气引流的。因此，这个区域是引起慢性鼻窦炎的关键部位。

诊断评估

鼻内镜检查：有慢性鼻窦炎病史的患者应在局麻下行硬内镜检查。特别要注意中鼻道的病变情况（图88），如有无息肉、脓性分泌物（图89）或某些阻碍鼻窦通气引流的异常解剖结构。
冠位CT扫描：当需行鼻内镜手术时，冠位CT可显示鼻窦的解剖（图90）、病变范围（图91）及其与毗邻结构（如眶内容物和前颅窝）的关系。

鼻内镜手术

慢性鼻窦炎经规范的药物治疗仍未治愈者，应采取鼻内镜手术。手术目的是清除鼻窦的病变黏膜，改善中鼻道区域的通气引流。通常行前组筛窦切除术，但如果病变范围广，累及后组筛窦和蝶窦，可行全组鼻窦开放术。

25 Functional endoscopic sinus surgery

The widespread availability of endoscopes and high-quality radiology has led to a reappraisal of many of the established methods of treatment for chronic sinusitis. Most sinus infections are rhinogenic, spreading from the nose into the sinuses. Both the frontal and maxillary sinuses are drained and ventilated through the narrow clefts of the anterior ethmoid cells, close to the middle nasal turbinate. It is this small area that is critical in the development of chronic sinusitis.

Diagnostic evaluation

Patients with a history suggestive of chronic sinusitis are evaluated by rigid endoscopy under local anaesthetic. The middle meatus is particularly important (Fig. 88), and is inspected for evidence of polyps, purulent secretion (Fig. 89) or anatomical abnormality that may impede sinus ventilation.

Where endoscopic surgery is necessary a CT scan in the coronal plane is obtained to show the underlying sinus anatomy (Fig. 90), the extent of chronic sinus disease (Fig. 91) and its relationship to adjacent structures such as the orbital contents and anterior cranial fossa.

Endoscopic surgery

When chronic sinusitis persists despite adequate medical treatment, patients may undergo endoscopic surgery. These operations remove diseased sinus mucosa and improve ventilation in the middle meatus area. Usually anterior ethmoidectomy is performed, but in more extensive disease access to the posterior ethmoidal and sphenoidal sinuses is possible.

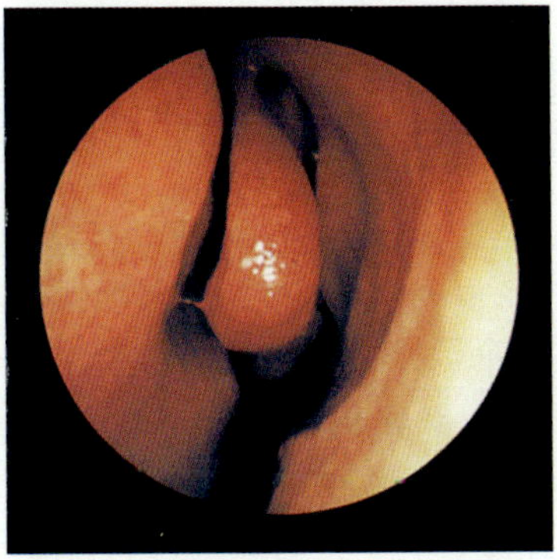

图 88　正常中鼻道
Normal middle meatus.

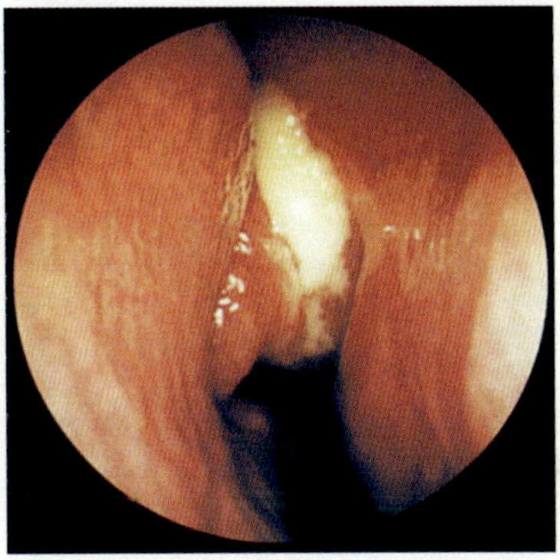

图 89　中鼻道脓液
Pus in the middle meatus.

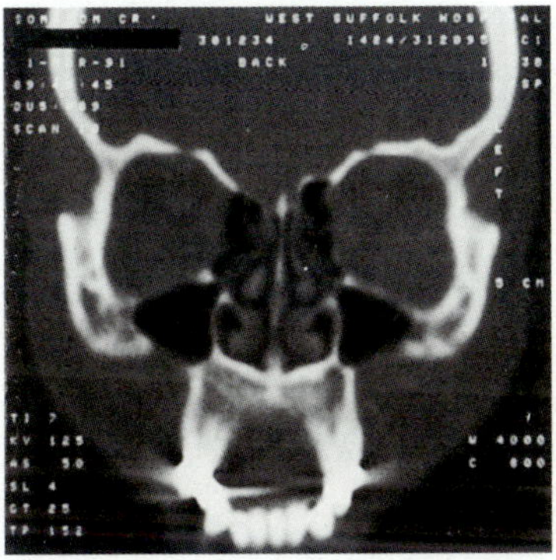

图 90　正常冠位 CT
Normal coronal CT scan.

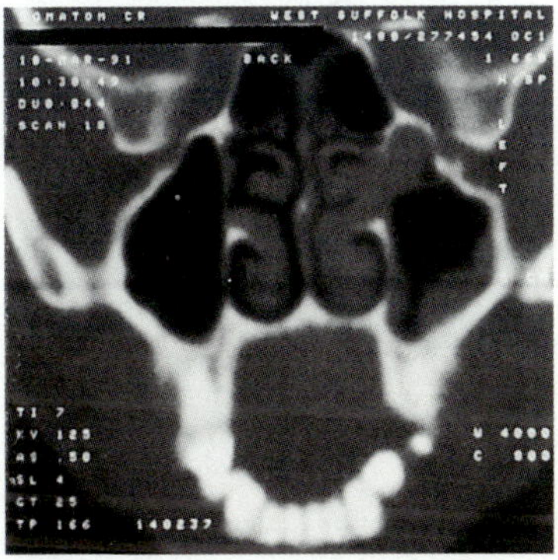

图 91　CT 显示筛窦病变
CT scan with ethmoidal disease.

26 腺样体

腺样体发生于鼻咽顶及鼻咽后壁的连接处，做为咽淋巴环的一部分而参与人体的体液免疫。出生时即存在，持续于整个童年时期，青春期后开始萎缩。

临床特征　腺样体肥大（图 92）阻塞鼻咽部气流，妨碍咽鼓管的开放，同时也成为邻近组织感染的病灶。临床多表现为：鼻堵、流涕、中耳渗出引起的听力下降以及反复中耳炎引起的耳痛。腺样体肥大多伴有扁桃体肥大，可引起睡眠呼吸暂停同时伴有白天嗜睡的症状。严重病例可引起肺动脉高压和肺源性心脏病，临床疑似病例可由鼻咽侧位片（图 93）确诊。

治疗　腺样体肥大引起的睡眠呼吸暂停、鼻堵或持续性中耳渗出性病变以及反复中耳炎者可行手术切除。

Adenoids 26

Lymphoid tissue found at the junction of the roof and posterior wall of the nasopharynx, thought to be involved in the development of humoral immunity as a component of the 'gut-associated lymphoid tissue' (GALT). Adenoid tissue is present at birth and during childhood, beginning to atrophy before puberty.

Clinical features

Adenoidal hypertrophy (Fig. 92) disturbs nasopharyngeal airflow and Eustachian tube function and can also act as a focus of infection for adjacent sites. Common clinical features are nasal obstruction and discharge, deafness due to middle ear effusion and otalgia due to recurrent otitis media. Gross adenoidal enlargement, often associated with tonsillar hypertrophy, can cause sleep apnoea syndrome in which apnoeic episodes during sleep are associated with daytime somnolence and in severe cases pulmonary hypertension and cor pulmonale. Clinical suspicion of enlarged adenoids can be confirmed by lateral radiography (Fig. 93).

Management

Surgical removal (adenoidectomy) can be undertaken if enlarged adenoids are causing sleep apnoea, nasal obstruction or are a contributing factor to persistent middle ear effusions or recurrent otitis media.

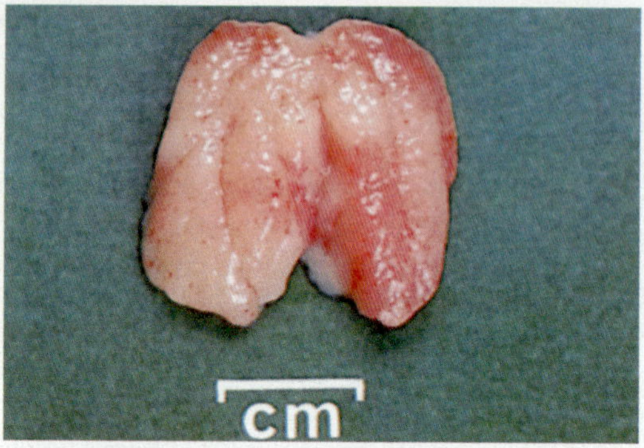

图 92　腺样体切除术后标本
Operative specimen of adenoids.

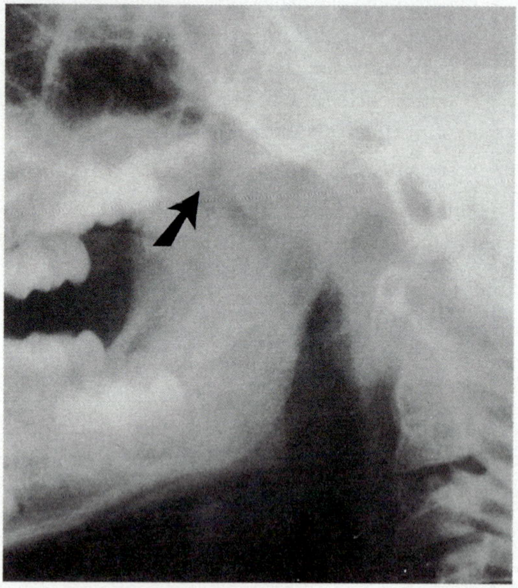

图 93　箭头所指为腺样体肥大
Adenoidal hypertrophy (arrowed).

面部骨折

鼻骨骨折

临床特征 该类型的骨折最为常见，能造成可触及的外鼻畸形（图 94）和鼻内损伤，例如中隔血肿或中隔偏曲。若筛窦受损可引起脑脊液鼻漏。

治疗 全麻或局麻下行鼻骨骨折复位。鼻中隔偏曲者可于Ⅱ期行黏膜下中隔切除术。

颧骨骨折

临床特征 通常为开放性骨折（图 95），常有面颊轮廓扁平和牙关紧闭。眶底受累常伴有眼球运动受限。

治疗 颧骨抬高复位术（常采用 Gillies 入路），并经柯 - 陆式入路行骨折复位内固定和上颌窦填塞。

上颌骨骨折

上颌骨骨折可按 Le Fort 分型分为 3 型（图 96）：

- Ⅰ型
- Ⅱ型
- Ⅲ型

临床特征 断离的骨碎片引起的呼吸道梗阻是危及生命的急症，错位咬合最为常见。

治疗 以弓形板固定游离骨片以及钢丝悬吊固定于双侧额骨或顶骨。

Facial fractures

Nasal fractures

Clinical features

This common fracture can produce an external deformity (Fig. 94) which may be palpable, and internal disruption, e.g. septal haematoma or septal deviation. Ethmoid involvement may produce CSF rhinorrhoea.

Management

Reduce any external bony deviation under general or local anaesthesia. A septal deviation may require a submucosal resection at a later date.

Zygomatic (malar) fractures

Clinical features

Usually tripartite (Fig. 95), the cheek contour is flattened and trismus is common. Orbital movements may be limited if the orbital floor is involved.

Management

Elevation of the zygoma (via a Gillies approach) may need to be supplemented by internal wiring and antral packing, through a Caldwell-Luc approach.

Maxillary (Le Fort) fractures

There are three types of maxillary or Le Fort fracture (Fig. 96):

- Type Ⅰ
- Type Ⅱ
- Type Ⅲ.

Clinical features

Airways obstruction by the mobile bone fragment is a serious threat. Malocclusion is common.

Management

Treatment involves fixing the mobile portion using arch bars and, frequently, bilateral suspension wiring from the frontal or parietal bones.

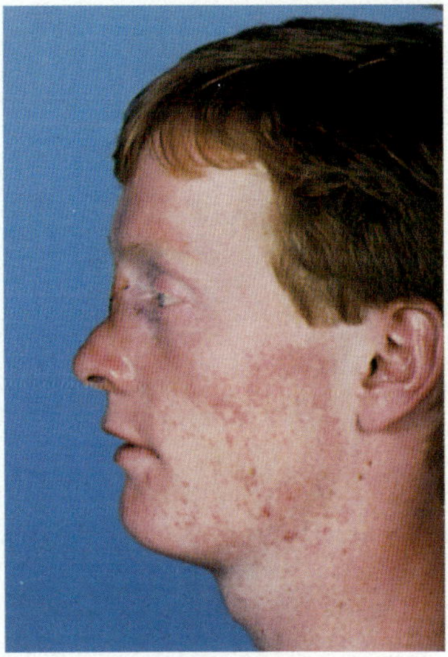

图 94　鼻骨骨折
Fractured nasal bones.

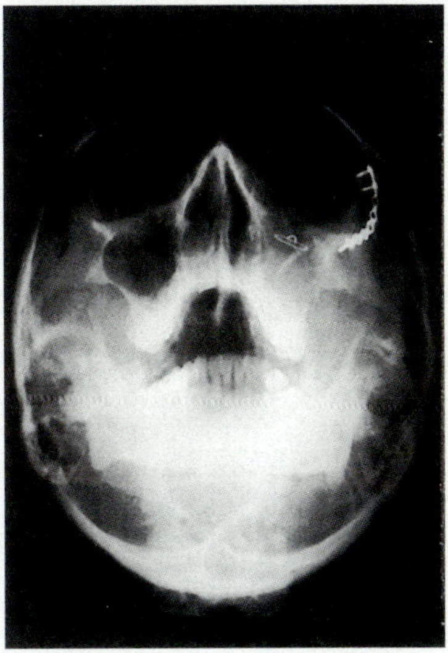

图 95　颧骨骨折切开复位术后
Zygomatic fracture after open reduction.

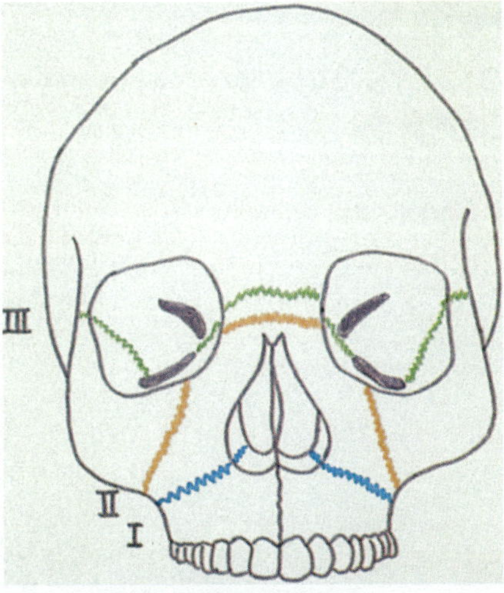

图 96　Le Fort 骨折分型
Types of Le Fort maxillary fractures.

28 鼻咽部肿瘤

鼻咽血管纤维瘤

发病率 为良性的血管肿瘤，常见于 25 岁以下的男性。

临床特征 常见症状有：鼻堵、鼻出血、中耳渗出引起的耳聋。

治疗 辅以术前 CT 扫描（图 97）、动脉血管造影及栓塞术的手术切除（图 98）。

恶性肿瘤

发病率 东南亚多见，占当地全身恶性肿瘤总数的 20%。

临床特征 表现为鼻堵、鼻出血、耳聋。颈淋巴结的转移可发生在局部症状出现之前。晚期病例可有脑神经麻痹的症状。

病理学 多为鳞癌，亦可见未分化癌及淋巴瘤。

治疗 活检病理确诊后放射治疗（图 99），手术治疗仅适用于放疗不敏感的颈淋巴结的处理。

脊索瘤

一种非常少见的发生于胚胎期颅底脊索残留的局部侵犯性的肿瘤。常表现为神经侵犯、鼻部和眼部症状。

Tumours of the nasopharynx 28

Angiofibroma

Incidence A benign vascular tumour occurring in males under the age of 25 years.

Clinical features Nasal obstruction, epistaxis and deafness due to middle ear effusion are common characteristics.

Management Treatment is by surgical excision, facilitated by preoperative CT scanning (Fig. 97), arteriography and embolization (Fig. 98).

Malignant tumours

Incidence Common in south east Asia, where they account for 20% of all malignant tumours.

Clinical features Present as nasal obstruction, epistaxis and deafness. Metastasis to cervical nodes may occur prior to local symptoms becoming apparent. Cranial nerve palsies occur in advanced cases.

Pathology Most are squamous carcinomas, although anaplastic carcinomas and lymphomas also occur.

Management Radiotherapy following biopsy confirmation (Fig. 99), with surgery used only for cervical nodes not responding to irradiation.

Chordoma

A very rare locally invasive neoplasm arising from remnants of the fetal notochord found in the skull base. Presents with neurological, nasal and ophthalmic symptoms.

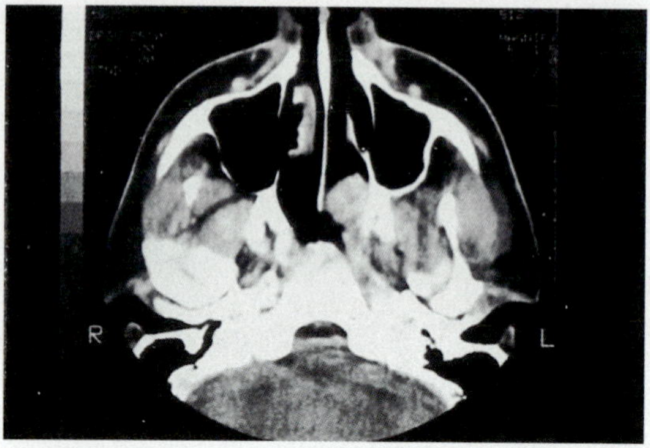

图 97 CT 显示的血管纤维瘤
CT scan showing an angiofibroma.

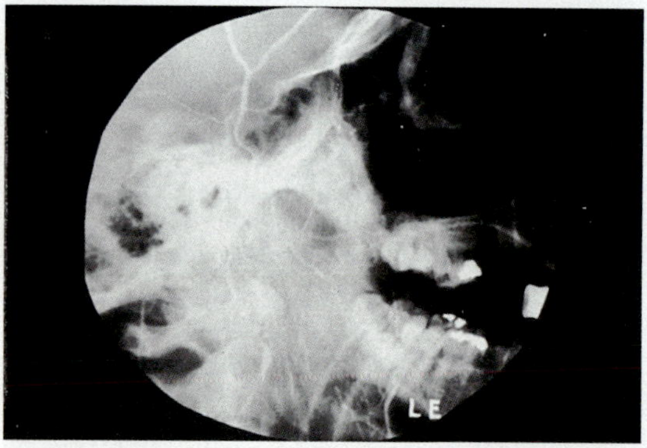

图 98 动脉血管造影显示血管纤维瘤的多血管状态
Arteriogram demonstrating vascularity of angiofibroma.

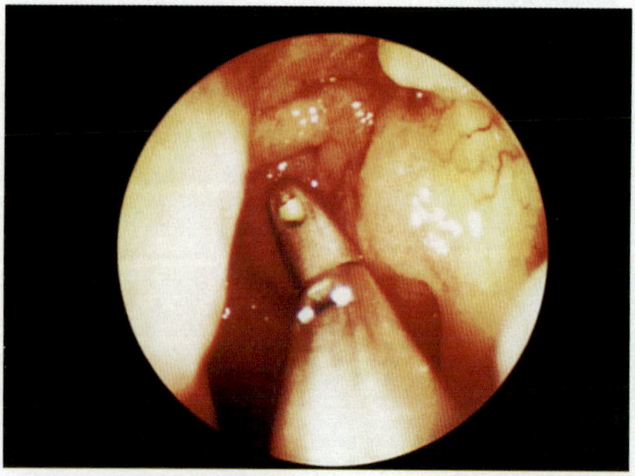

图 99 鼻咽癌内镜下活检
Endoscopic biopsy of a nasopharyngeal carcinoma.

鼻窦肿瘤

病理学

良性肿瘤：包括乳头状瘤、腺瘤、骨瘤以及血管瘤。内翻性乳头状瘤可发生恶变。

恶性肿瘤：50% 的恶性肿瘤见于上颌窦。最常见的类型为鳞癌，其他的还有腺癌、腺样囊性癌、黑色素瘤以及肉瘤。

临床特征

良性肿瘤多表现为单侧的息肉样肿物。恶性肿瘤向中线发展可有鼻堵、鼻出血，向后可有咽鼓管阻塞和脑神经麻痹的症状，向下可侵犯牙齿（图 100），向上可造成突眼或溢泪，向侧面可引起面颊的肿胀。

治疗

治疗前需行组织学诊断以及应用CT鼻窦断层扫描等影像学手段明确肿瘤的范围（图 101）。良性肿瘤可予以局部切除，经内镜下或鼻外侧切开入路。恶性肿瘤预后不良，多由于临床发现较晚，且多广泛侵犯。若有根治的可能可行根治性切除（上颌骨切除术）联合放疗的综合治疗，术后可用齿板和赝复体行术后颌面缺损的修复（图 102）。

29 Paranasal sinus tumours

Pathology

Benign tumours: include papillomas, adenomas, osteomas and angiomas. The inverting papilloma may undergo malignant change.

Malignant tumours: 50% of malignant tumours are found in the maxillary sinus. Squamous cell carcinoma is the most common type. Others include adenocarcinoma, adenoid cystic carcinoma, melanoma and sarcoma.

Clinical features

Benign tumours frequently present as a unilateral nasal polyp. Malignant tumours spread medially to produce nasal obstruction or epistaxis, posteriorly to give Eustachian tube obstruction and cranial nerve palsies, inferiorly to disrupt the teeth (Fig. 100) or superiorly to give proptosis or epiphora. Lateral spread produces swelling of the cheek.

Management

Prior to treatment planning, histological diagnosis and radiological assessment of the extent of the tumour using CT scanning and sinus tomography are necessary (Fig.101). Benign tumours are treated by local excision, either endoscopically or by an external lateral rhinotomy approach. Malignant tumours have a poor prognosis due to their late presentation and extensive spread. When curative treatment is possible a combination of radical surgery (maxillectomy) and radiotherapy is usually used. The resulting defect is filled with a dental plate and obturator (Fig.102).

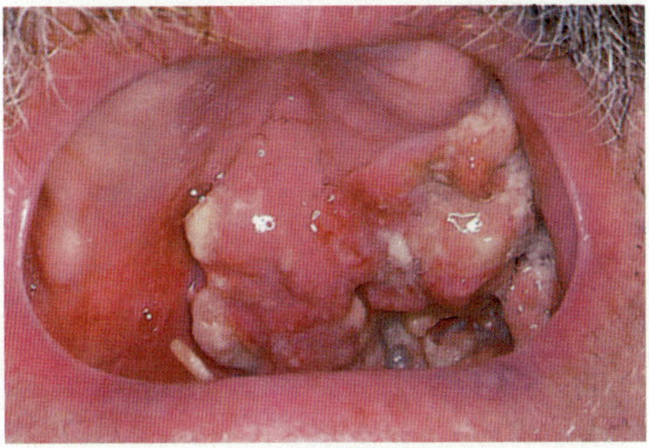

图 100　鼻窦恶性肿瘤侵犯硬腭
Antral carcinoma involving hard palate.

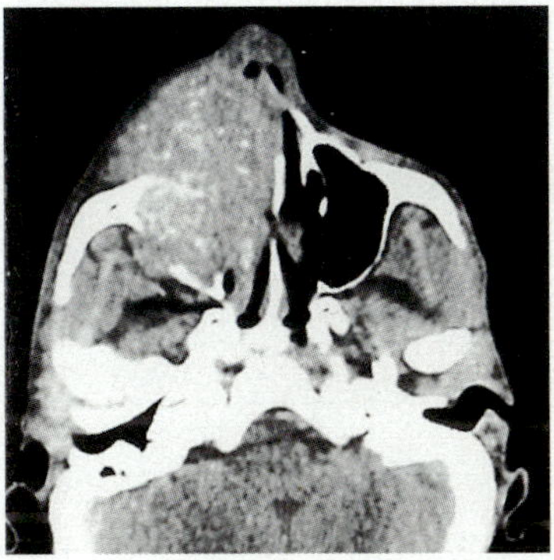

图 101　CT 显示鼻窦癌的范围
Extensive antral carcinoma on CT scan.

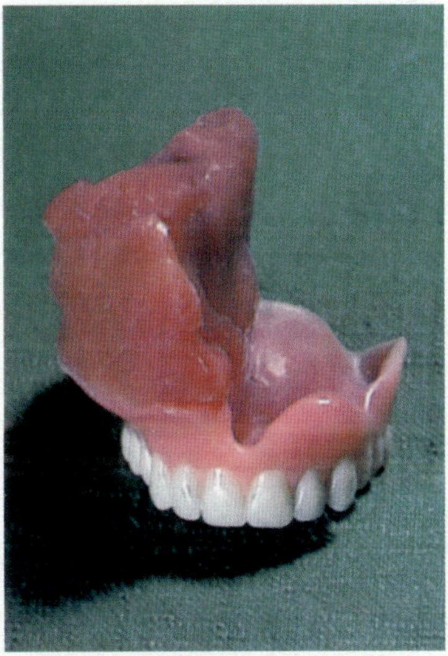

图 102　齿板和赝复体
Dental plate and obturator.

30 儿童鼻气道阻塞

儿童的鼻堵常由其父母发现，尤其在伴有流涕和打鼾时。腺样体肥大是引起小儿鼻堵最主要的原因，但以下情况仍应引起注意。

后鼻孔闭锁

病因 胚胎时的鼻颊膜残留引起先天性鼻后孔闭锁。闭锁多发生于鼻后部近硬腭缘。

临床特征 双侧鼻后孔闭锁表现为出生时的呼吸困难，由于必经口呼吸，喂养时呼吸困难加重。单侧的病例症状表现较晚，多有单侧的鼻堵、流涕。由鼻腔插入橡皮导管，观察其不能通过鼻腔到达咽部而诊断，亦可由CT检查确诊（图 103）。

治疗 经由鼻腔或硬腭的闭锁板的切除。

鼻腔异物

多见于儿童，常见的有：小珠、海绵条或纸片等（图 104）。

临床特征 常表现为单侧涕中带血、鼻前庭炎、鼻内恶臭。

治疗 不能配合的小儿可行全麻下异物取出。

Nasal airway obstruction in children

Nasal obstruction in children is usually noted by parents, particularly when accompanied by rhinorrhoea and snoring. Adenoid hypertrophy is the most common cause of paediatric nasal obstruction; however, the following conditions should also be borne in mind.

Posterior choanal atresia

Aetiology

A congenital condition caused by persistence of the embryonic bucconasal membrane. The obstruction is at the posterior end of the nose near the edge of the hard palate.

Clinical features

In bilateral cases there is respiratory difficulty at birth aggravated by feeding and necessitating the use of an oral airway. Unilateral cases present later with unilateral nasal obstruction and rhinorrhoea. Diagnosis is made by the inability to pass a rubber catheter through the nose into the pharynx and is confirmed by CT scanning (Fig. 103).

Management

Surgical division of the atretic plate by the transnasal or transpalatal route is required.

Nasal foreign body

A common occurrence in children, e.g. with beads, pieces of sponge or paper (Fig. 104).

Clinical features

Typically presents with unilateral foul blood-stained rhinorrhoea, nasal vestibulitis and fetor.

Management

A general anaesthetic is occasionally required for removal in an uncooperative child.

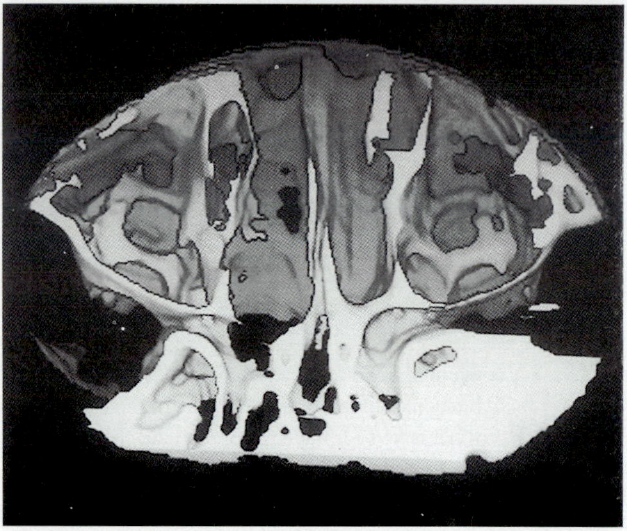

图 103　鼻后孔闭锁（三维重建）
Choanal atresia (3D reconstruction).

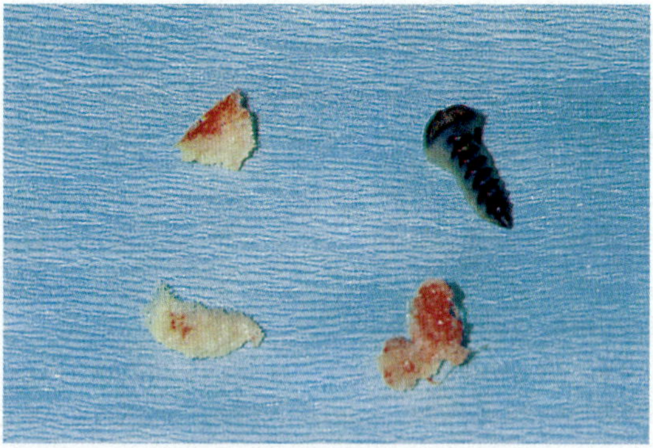

图 104　某患儿鼻腔内异物
Foreign bodies removed from a child's nose.

儿童喉阻塞

临床特征　喉喘鸣是喉梗阻的特征性表现。吸气性喉喘鸣表明声门或声门上区的梗阻，呼气性喉喘鸣表明支气管梗阻，双向性喉喘鸣表明声门下区梗阻。若喉喘鸣伴有发绀、心动过速、肋间隙和胸骨窝的塌陷（图105），必须急救手术处理以挽救生命。不甚严重的病例可出现声嘶、喂养困难和反复的肺部感染。

先天性喉阻塞

病因　先天性异常包括：喉囊肿、喉蹼、喉狭窄、血管环以及声带麻痹。喉软骨软化病是由喉软骨过度软化引起声门上框架于吸气相垂入气道而引起梗阻，随年龄增大而自愈。

治疗　任何先天性喉喘鸣均需行直接喉镜检查。

后天性喉阻塞

病因　急性会厌炎：由流感嗜血杆菌感染引起，可导致急性进行性气道梗阻（图106）。

急性喉气管支气管炎（哮吼）：由副流感病毒或呼吸道合胞病毒感染引起的喉、气管、支气管的水肿、渗出、结痂。

声门下狭窄：多由婴儿气管切开或长时间的气管内插管引起。

治疗　急性会厌炎：静脉用氯霉素，必要时气管内插管或紧急气管切开。

急性喉气管支气管炎：很少病例需气管内插管。

31 Laryngeal obstruction in children

Clinical features

The hallmark of laryngeal obstruction is stridor. Inspiratory stridor indicates glottic or supraglottic obstruction, expiratory stridor bronchial obstruction and two-way stridor subglottic obstruction. If stridor is accompanied by cyanosis, tachycardia and intercostal and sternal recession (Fig.105), urgent measures are needed to save life. In less severe cases a hoarse voice, feeding problems and recurrent chest infections may occur.

Congenital laryngeal obstruction

Aetiology

Congenital anomalies include laryngeal cysts, webs, stenosis, vascular rings and vocal cord paralysis. Laryngomalacia is a condition caused by abnormal flaccidity of the larynx allowing the supraglottic structures to be drawn into the airway on inspiration; the condition resolves with age.

Management

All cases of congenital stridor should undergo direct laryngoscopy.

Acquired laryngeal obstruction

Aetiology

Acute epiglottitis: due to *Haemophilus influenzae.* It causes rapidly progressive airway obstruction (Fig. 106).

Acute laryngotracheobronchitis (croup): due to para-influenzae virus or respiratory syncytial virus. It produces oedema, exudates and crusting of the larynx, trachea and bronchi.

Subglottic stenosis: may follow infant tracheostomy or prolonged endotracheal intubation.

Management

Acute epiglottitis: treatment is with intravenous chloramphenicol. Endotracheal intubation or an emergency tracheostomy may be necessary.

Acute laryngotracheobronchitis: endotracheal intubation is rarely required.

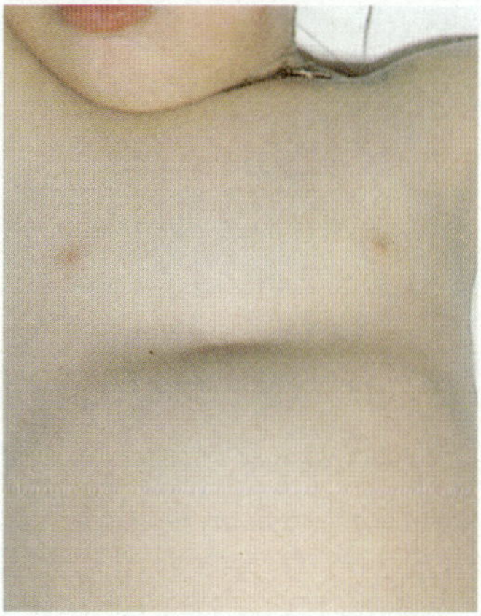

图 105 小儿上呼吸道梗阻的吸气相胸骨内陷
Sternal recession in a child with upper airways obstruction.

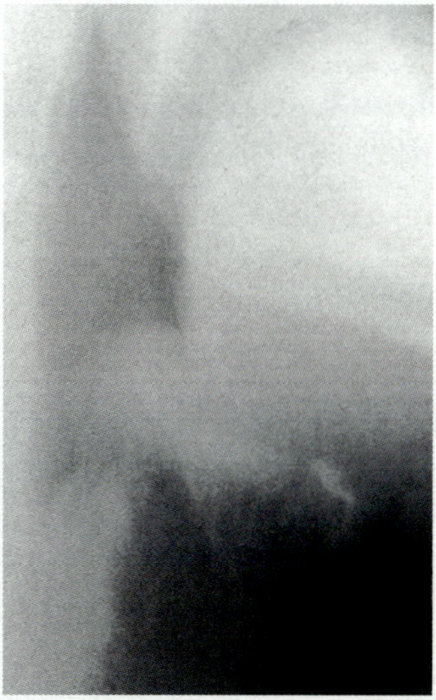

图 106 急性会厌炎的会厌肿胀
Epiglottic swelling in acute epiglottitis.

32 急性扁桃体炎

发病率 是耳鼻咽喉科非常常见的疾病，特别多发于 4 ~ 10 岁的儿童。

病因 超过 50% 的病例由乙型溶血性链球菌感染引起，另可见病毒、葡萄球菌、肺炎球菌感染。

临床特征 咽痛、吞咽困难、吞咽痛、耳痛以及发热、全身不适等症。咽腔黏膜充血、扁桃体肿大伴脓点及脓液渗出（图 107）。反复感染后可引起扁桃体慢性增大（图 108）。淋巴结炎多见于颈内静脉二腹肌淋巴结。全血细胞计数显示白细胞增多，但细菌培养不一定能有阳性结果。

鉴别诊断 *感染性单核细胞增多症*：可由嗜异性凝集试验和血象结果（此症有非典型单核细胞和淋巴细胞增多）鉴别。

恶性血液病：任何原因导致的白细胞异常均可引起免疫功能受损，继而患者表现为严重的咽炎，例如：急性白血病。

白喉：少见，但若扁桃体表面有膜性渗出或严重的呼吸道梗阻时应特别注意。

Acute tonsillitis

Incidence

A very common disease particularly affecting children between the ages of 4 and 10 years.

Aetiology

Over 50% of the cases are due to a B haemolytic streptococcus, the majority of the others being of viral, staphylococcal or pneumococcal origin.

Clinical features

Sore throat, dysphagia, pain on swallowing and otalgia are associated with pyrexia and general malaise. The pharyngeal mucosa appears red and the tonsils are often enlarged and covered by discrete microabscesses or a confluent exudate (Fig. 107). The tonsils often remain chronically enlarged and inflamed (Fig. 108). Lymphadenopathy is frequent, the jugulo-digastric nodes being most commonly involved. A full blood count reveals a leukocytosis but a bacteriology swab does not always grow the pathogen concerned.

Differential diagnosis

Infectious mononucleosis. It may be impossible to distinguish between the two without a Paul-Bunnell test and a differential white cell count (the latter shows atypical monocytes and a lymphocytosis).

Blood dyscrasias. Any white cell abnormality giving an impaired immune status may present as a severe pharyngitis, e.g. acute leukaemia.

Diphtheria. Rarely seen but should always be borne in mind when there is a membranous exudate over the tonsils or when severe airways obstruction is evident.

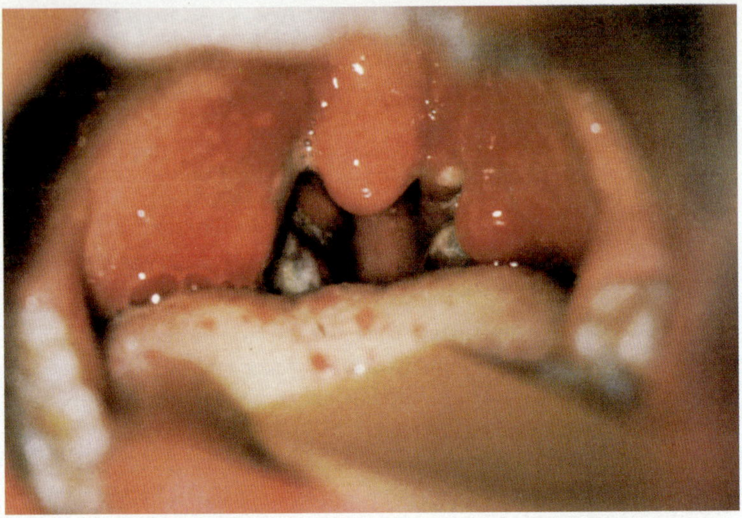

图 107　急性渗出性扁桃体炎
Acute exudative tonsillitis.

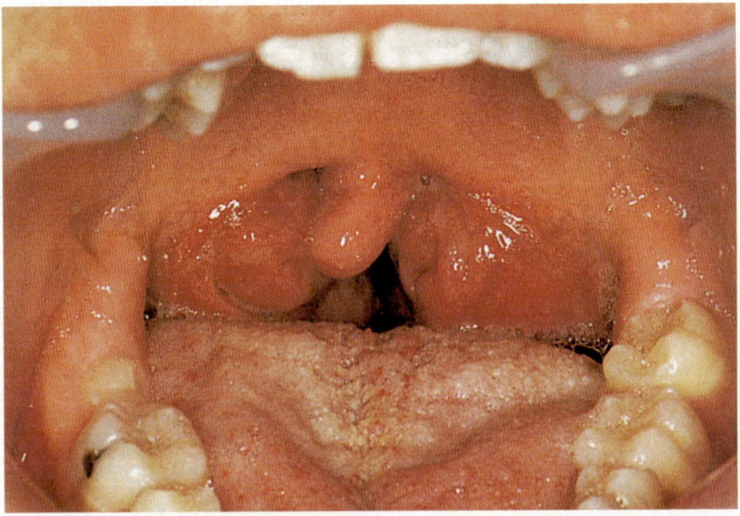

图 108　反复感染后扁桃体慢性增大
Chronically enlarged tonsils following recurrent infection.

治疗

卧床休息、抗生素和适当补液。无青霉素过敏或药敏试验显示细菌耐药者均需静脉或口服青霉素。扁桃体肿大引起呼吸道梗阻的重症患者可行气管切开。

长期反复发作的扁桃体炎可行扁桃体切除术（图109）。术后扁桃体窝有7～10天的愈合期，期间用白膜覆盖（图110），类似溃疡性咽炎。此间可有继发性的出血和感染。

并发症

- 慢性扁桃体炎；
- 扁桃体周脓肿（扁周脓肿）（图111）：住院治疗，抗生素及经口切开引流；
- 咽旁脓肿：需颈外入路切开引流；
- 急性中耳炎；
- 链球菌感染后风湿热 / 肾小球肾炎：已少见。

Management

Bed rest, antibiotics and adequate hydration. Penicillin is given (orally or intravenously) unless organism sensitivities or allergy dictate otherwise. In severe cases with grossly enlarged tonsils a tracheostomy may be necessary for airways obstruction.

Recurrent episodes over a prolonged period of time are best managed by tonsillectomy (Fig. 109). Following surgery the tonsillar fossae heal over a period of 7-10 days during which time they are covered by a slough (Fig. 110), which may mimic an ulcerative pharyngitis. Infection and secondary haemorrhage from the fossae can occur during this period.

Complications

- Chronic tonsillitis
- Peritonsillar abscess (quinsy) (Fig. 111): hospitalization, antibiotics and intraoral incision and drainage are required
- Parapharyngeal abscess: requires surgical drainage through an external neck incision
- Acute otitis media
- Post-streptococcal rheumatic fever/glomerulonephritis: now rare.

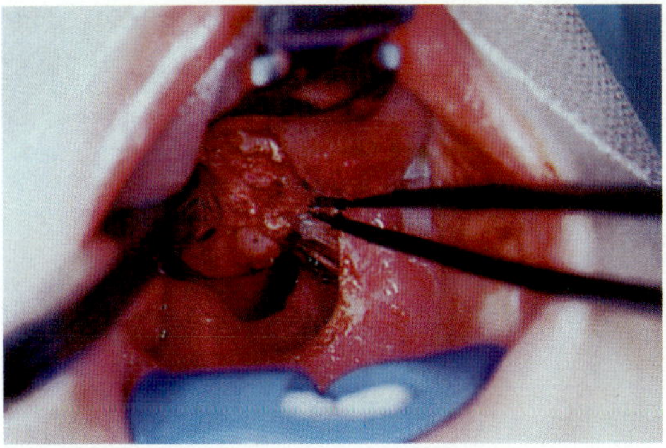

图 109　双极电刀扁桃体切除术
Dissection tonsillectomy using bipolar diathermy.

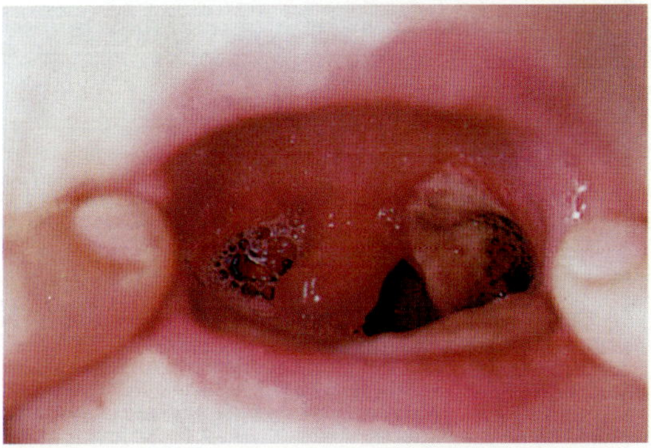

图 110　扁桃体切除术后覆盖扁桃体窝的假膜
Post-tonsillectomy slough overlying tonsillar fossae.

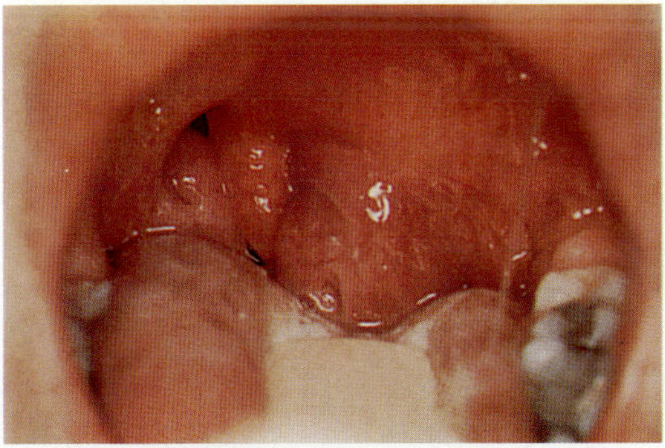

图 111　左侧扁桃体周脓肿
Left-sided quinsy.

33 颈部间隙感染

急性咽后脓肿

多由小儿急性上呼吸道感染后咽后淋巴结炎引起。

临床特征 表现为：咽痛、发热、咽后壁肿胀。侧位 X 线片可见咽后间隙组织肿胀（图 112）。

治疗 脓肿需经口引流，且要注意防范误吸。

慢性咽后脓肿

多由成人颈椎结核引起。

临床特征 咽后壁正中部肿胀，X 线示颈椎疾病。

治疗 抗结核化学治疗。

咽旁脓肿

咽旁间隙感染可由扁桃体感染或下列第三磨牙感染引起。

临床特征 咽痛，牙关紧闭。扁桃体被推向中线伴颈部肿胀（图 113）。

治疗 在足量的抗生素治疗下可行颈外入路切开引流。

Ludwig 咽峡炎

临床特征 继发于牙病或扁桃体炎的下颌下间隙蜂窝织炎，表现为颏下区（图 114）和口底的肿胀。

治疗 大剂量抗生素治疗。

Acute retropharyngeal abscess

Lymphadenitis of the retropharyngeal nodes following an upper respiratory tract infection in children.

Clinical features Presents with sore throat, pyrexia and swelling of the posterior pharyngeal wall. Lateral X-ray shows retropharyngeal swelling (Fig. 112).

Management The abscess should be drained via the mouth with precautions taken to avoid inhalation of pus.

Chronic retropharyngeal abscess

Occurs in adults in association with tuberculous cervical spine disease.

Clinical features Swelling is seen in the midline of the pharynx and X-rays show vertebral disease.

Management Treatment is with antituberculous chemotherapy.

Parapharyngeal abscess

The tissue space lateral to the pharynx may become infected by spread of organisms from the tonsils or lower third molar teeth.

Clinical features Presents with sore throat and trismus. The tonsil is pushed medially and there is neck swelling (Fig. 113).

Management Treatment is by incision and drainage via the neck followed by appropriate antibiotic therapy.

Ludwig's angina

Clinical features Cellulitis of the submandibular space secondary to dental disease or tonsillitis presents with swelling of the submental region (Fig. 114) and floor of the mouth.

Management Treat with high-dose antibiotics.

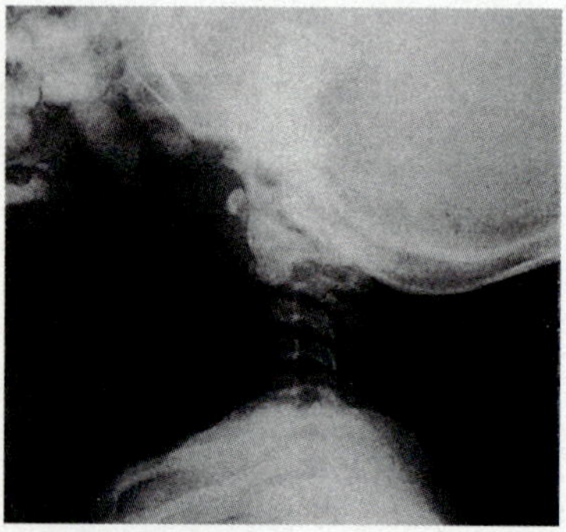

图 112　咽后脓肿
Retropharyngeal abscess.

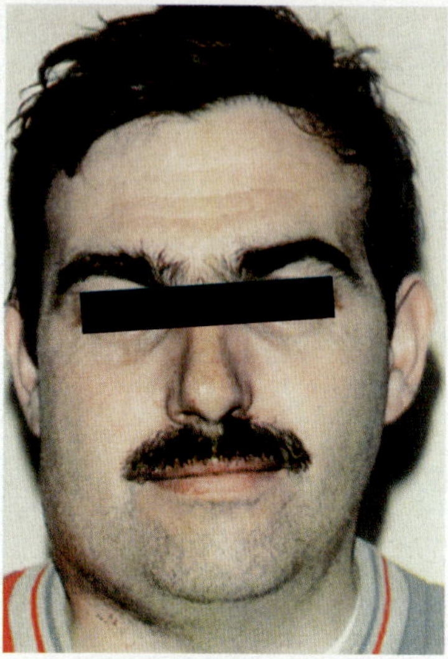

图 113　咽旁脓肿
Parapharyngeal abscess.

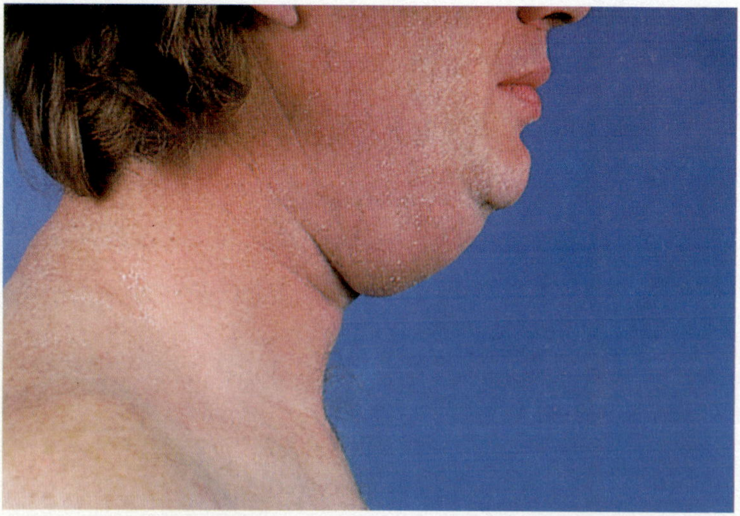

图 114　Ludwig 咽峡炎
Ludwig's angina.

舌良性疾病

舌甲状腺

病因 胚胎时，源于舌盲孔的组织向下凹陷并向颈部迁移形成甲状腺。甲状腺组织可见于下降路径中的任何部位，例如舌甲状腺（图 115）或甲状舌管囊肿。

临床特征 常表现为吞咽困难。出血和呼吸道梗阻少见。

治疗 若在颈其他部位能有功能正常的甲状腺组织，则引起症状的舌甲状腺可予以切除。

黑毛舌

病因 舌前部的丝状乳头过度增生并伴有黑或棕色外观（图 116）。

临床特征 可无其他症状，仅表现为颜色改变。

治疗 舌背的机械性刷刮。

地图舌

发病率 人群发病率为 1%。

临床特征 发生于舌背的不规则形状的舌乳头缺失（图 117）。大小、形状各异且随时间变化。

治疗 无需治疗。

34 Benign conditions of the tongue

Lingual thyroid

Aetiology

Tissue originating from the site of the foramen caecum invaginates and migrates down into the lower neck to form the thyroid gland. Thyroid tissue may be found at any point along this path of descent, e.g. lingual thyroid (Fig. 115) or thyroglossal cyst.

Clinical features

Usually presents as dysphagia. Haemorrhage and airway obstruction rarely occur.

Management

Once functioning thyroid tissue has been demonstrated elsewhere in the neck, the lump may be removed if it is causing significant symptoms.

Black hairy tongue

Aetiology

Caused by overgrowth and elongation of the filiform papillae of the anterior tongue in association with their black or brown discoloration (Fig. 116).

Clinical features

Asymptomatic, but for its appearance.

Management

Treatment is by mechanical brushing or scraping of the dorsum of the tongue.

Geographic tongue

Incidence

Affects 1% of the population.

Clinical features

Irregularly shaped areas of depapillation occur over the dorsum of the tongue (Fig. 117). The patches vary in size and distribution over a period of days.

Management

No treatment is required.

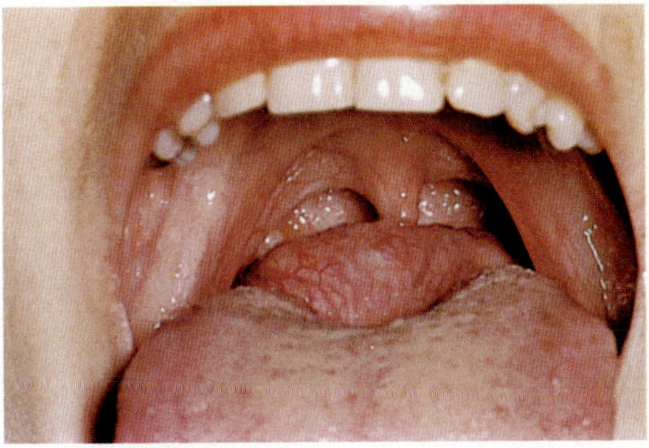

图 115　舌甲状腺
Lingual thyroid.

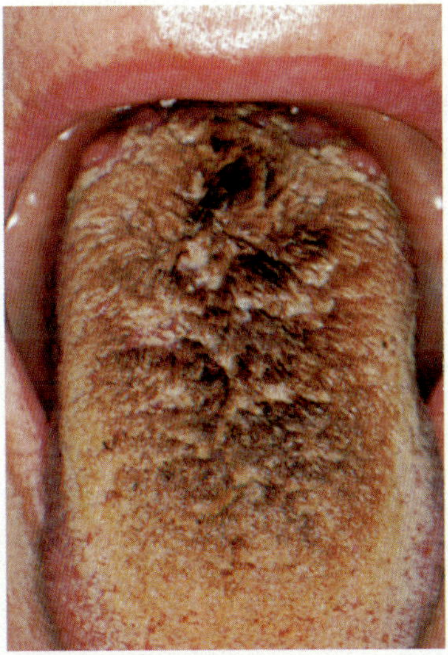

图 116　黑毛舌
Black hairy tongue.

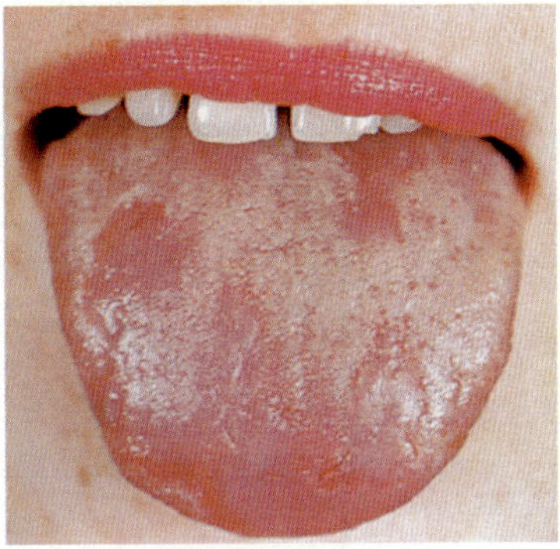

图 117　地图舌
Geographic tongue.

35 舌白斑和舌癌

白斑

仅表现为不可擦除的白色斑块（图 118）。口腔或舌白斑发生的危险因素包括：饮酒、吸烟、辛辣食物、槟榔、梅毒以及牙源性外伤。大约5%的恶变率，诊断时有必要排除与之相关的癌性病变。

舌癌

绝大部分为鳞癌，可无前期的白斑。

临床特征

可表现为舌部外生性或浸润性的包块（图 119）。疼痛和吞咽困难常见。反射性耳痛（经舌神经和舌咽神经）亦可发生。多数肿瘤直径＞ 2cm，且 50% 伴有可触及的淋巴结转移。

治疗

1．小型病损

放疗，应用外照射或间质植入技术（图 120）。或外科治疗，可行部分舌或半舌切除（图 121）。上述各种治疗方法疗效相当。

2．大型病损

单独放疗或手术治疗，或放疗结合手术治疗的综合治疗。以上治疗方法均造成口腔功能的障碍，特别是言语和吞咽功能的障碍。

Leukoplakia and tongue carcinoma

Leukoplakia

A white patch which cannot be wiped away and for which no other diagnosis is apparent (Fig. 118). Risk factors in the development of oral cavity or tongue leukoplakia include alcohol, smoking, spice and betel nut chewing, syphilis and dental trauma. About 5% of cases become malignant. Exclusion of an associated carcinoma is essential.

Tongue carcinoma

Almost all tongue carcinomas are squamous in origin. There need not be any pre-existing leukoplakia.

Clinical features

May present as an exophytic or infiltrative lump on the tongue (Fig. 119). Pain and dysphagia are common. Referred otalgia (via lingual and glossopharyngeal nerves) may also occur. At presentation most tumours are greater than 2cm diameter and 50% have palpably involved lymph nodes.

Management

Small lesions. Radiotherapy, using external beam or interstitial implant techniques (Fig. 120), or surgery, in the form of a partial or hemiglossectomy (Fig. 121) are equally effective.

Large lesions. Treatment is with radiotherapy or surgery alone or a planned combination of the two. Both modalities produce quite severe functional disability in the oral cavity, especially regarding speech and swallowing.

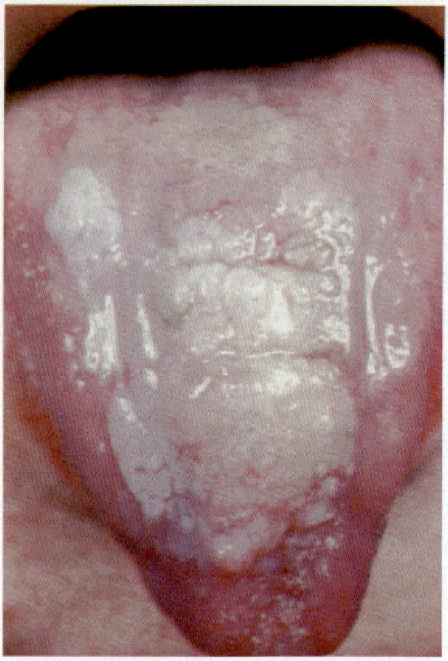

图 118　舌白斑
Leukoplakia of the tongue.

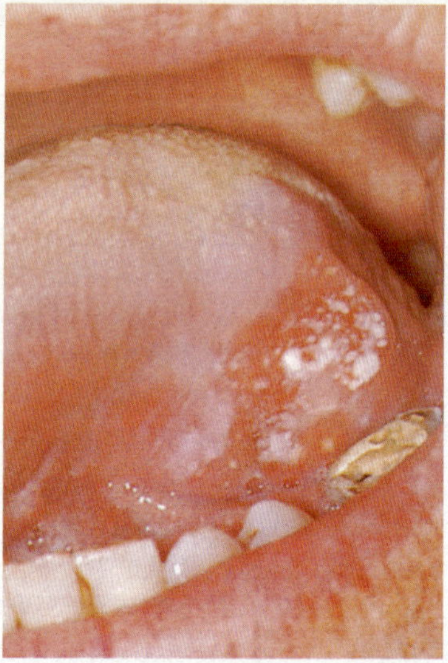

图 119　溃疡型舌癌
Ulcerative tongue carcinoma.

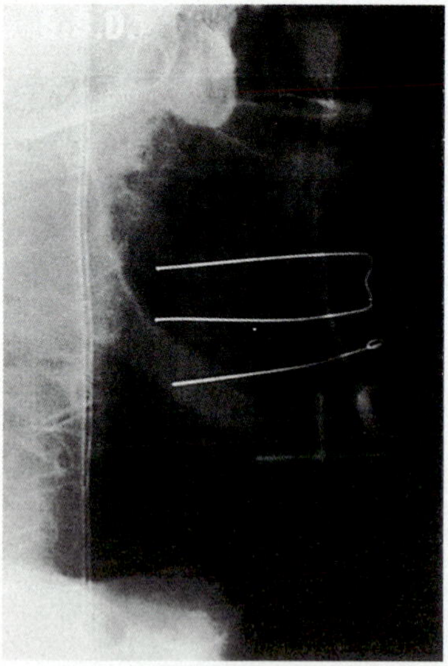

图 120　舌间质内植入物
Interstitial implant in the tongue.

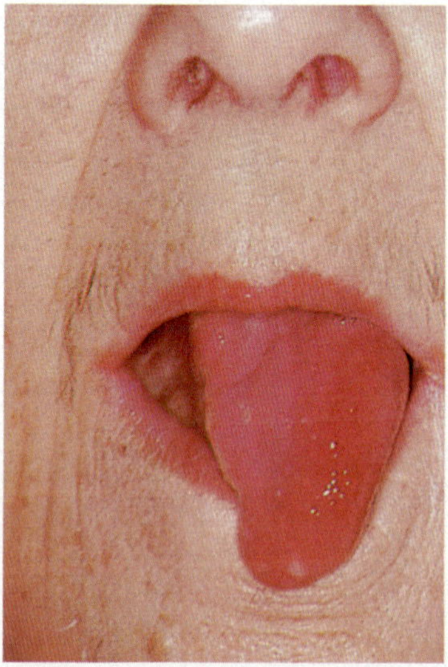

图 121　半舌切除术后
Tongue after hemiglossectomy.

扁桃体肿瘤

良性囊肿

临床特征 黏液潴留性囊肿、由扁桃体结石或聚集上皮碎片形成的囊肿常见。表面光滑，且位居于扁桃体的某一部位（图 122）。

治疗 症状性囊肿可行扁桃体切除。

淋巴瘤

临床特征 患侧扁桃体肥大、表面黏膜完整（图 123），可引起吞咽困难，此类患者应高度怀疑淋巴瘤。扁桃体橡皮样质感。切除后送病理活检可确诊。

治疗 限局性的病变可行局部放射治疗。晚期病例可加用化疗。

癌

临床特征 扁桃体鳞状细胞癌可表现为耳痛、咽痛或吞咽困难，多见于重度吸烟饮酒者。超过 50% 的患者伴有同侧颈淋巴结转移，这几乎是此类患者通常的就诊症状。检查时可见扁桃体坚硬且伴有溃疡（图 124）。

治疗 经过全面、细致的内镜和病理检查，原发灶较局限且无淋巴结转移者最适宜行放疗。手术（包括颈清扫术、下颌骨部分切除术和原发灶切除）仅适于放疗失败病例或原发灶过大者。

36 Tumours of the tonsil

Benign cysts

Clinical features Mucous retention cysts, tonsilloliths or cysts of inspissated epithelial debris may occur. They are smooth and localized to one portion of the tonsil (Fig. 122).

Management Symptomatic cysts may be helped by tonsillectomy.

Lymphoma

Clinical features Unilateral tonsillar swelling with an intact overlying mucosa (Fig. 123) may cause dysphagia and is suspicious of a lymphoma. The tonsil feels rubbery. Excision biopsy confirms the diagnosis.

Management After staging the disease, treatment involves radiotherapy for localized disease, with chemotherapy being added in more advanced cases.

Carcinoma

Clinical features Squamous carcinoma of the tonsil presents as otalgia, sore throat or dysphagia in heavy drinkers and smokers. More than 50% of cases have involved neck nodes ipsilaterally: this may be the mode of presentation. The tonsil is hard and ulcerated (Fig. 124).

Management After full endoscopy and biopsy small primaries without nodes are best treated by radiotherapy. Surgery (which involves a block dissection of neck, partial mandibulectomy and excision of the primary) is reserved for radiation failures and large primaries.

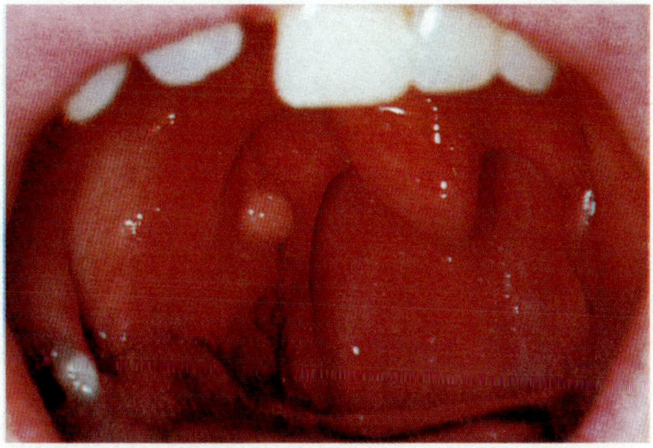

图 122　黏液潴留性囊肿
Tonsil retention cyst.

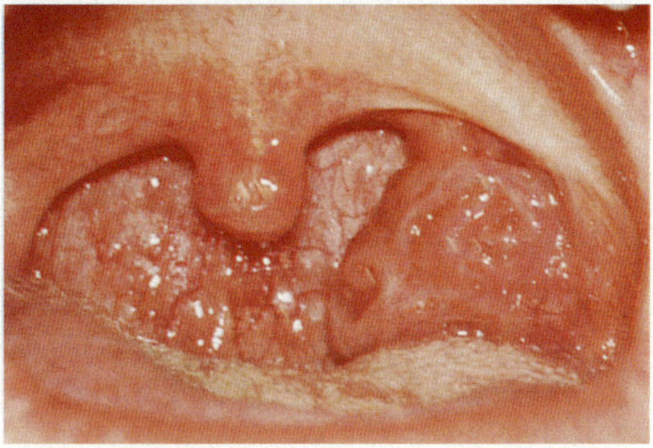

图 123　扁桃体淋巴瘤
Tonsil lymphoma.

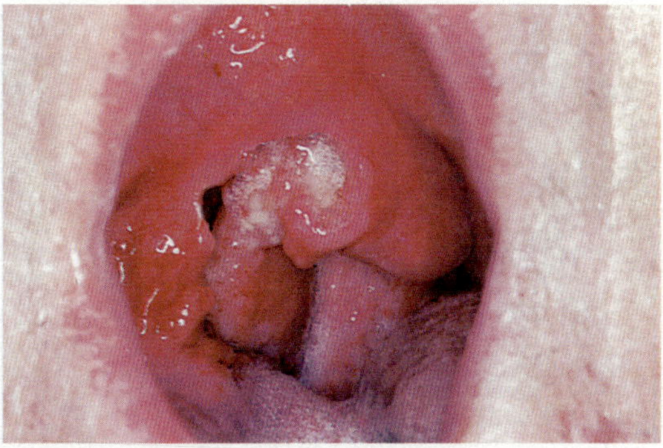

图 124　右扁桃体癌
Carcinoma of the right tonsil.

37 腭部疾病

腭隆凸

临床特征 表现为硬腭中线的单叶或多叶的骨性隆起（图 125）。病因未明。

治疗 若需安装假牙或肿胀影响进食，可将隆凸磨除。

硬腭肿瘤

虽多由上颌窦肿瘤向下侵犯而来，但仍可见硬腭原发的良、恶性肿瘤（图 126）。

临床特征 表现为：牙齿脱落、假牙托不适及面部肿胀。多形性腺瘤、腺样囊性癌、鳞癌最为常见。

治疗 依病理类型不同，可行手术切除和 / 或施行放疗。

腭裂和唇裂

两种最为常见的先天性异常。

临床特征 腭裂和唇裂可独立发生（图 127），但仍常伴发。最早表现为喂养障碍，而后可有面部发育障碍。腭裂常伴有因咽鼓管功能障碍而引起的中耳积液。

治疗 整形手术修复腭唇裂，术后需进行长期的牙列矫正，并筛查中耳有无积液。

Diseases of the palate

Torus palatinus

Clinical features

Presents as a unilobular or multilobular bony protruberance in the midline of the hard palate (Fig. 125). The aetiology is unknown.

Management

The torus can be reduced by drilling if a denture needs to be worn or if the swelling interferes with eating.

Palatal tumours

Although these are usually due to inferior extension of a maxillary sinus tumour, benign or malignant neoplasms can arise from the palate itself (Fig. 126).

Clinical features

Presents with loose teeth, ill-fitting dentures and facial swelling. The most common types are the pleomorphic adenoma, adenoid cystic carcinoma and squamous carcinoma.

Management

Treatment is by surgical excision and/or radiotherapy, depending on the histological diagnosis.

Clefts of the palate and lip

Two of the most common congenital anomalies.

Clinical features

Clefts of the lip and palate can occur in isolation (Fig. 127) but they often occur together. Initial difficulties may be encountered with feeding, with abnormal facial development later. Palatal clefts are often associated with middle ear effusions owing to Eustachian tube dysfunction.

Management

Plastic surgical repair of clefts with long-term orthodontic care and screening for middle ear effusions.

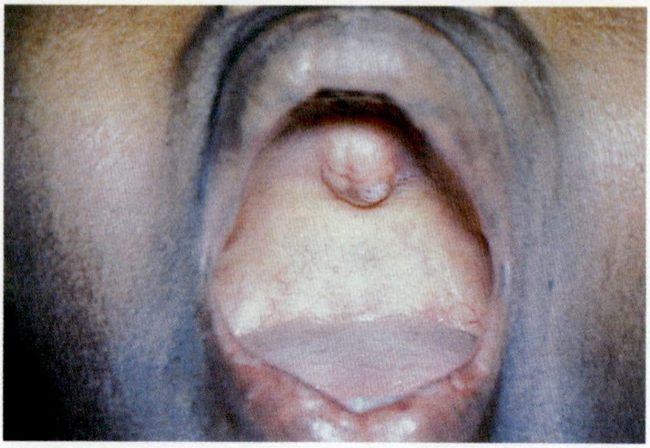

图 125　腭隆凸
Torus palatinus.

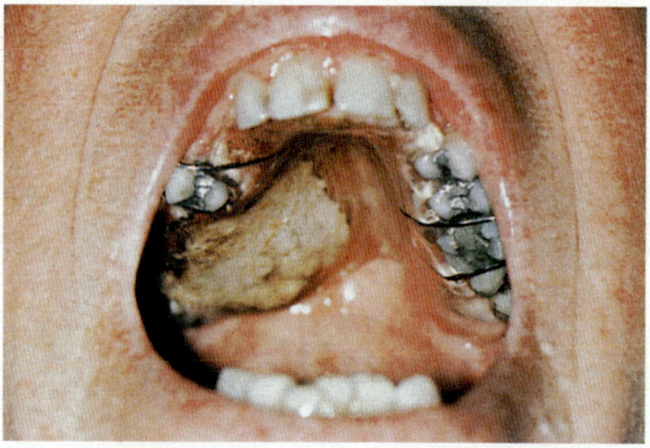

图 126　硬腭多形性腺瘤
Pleomorphic adenoma of the hard palate.

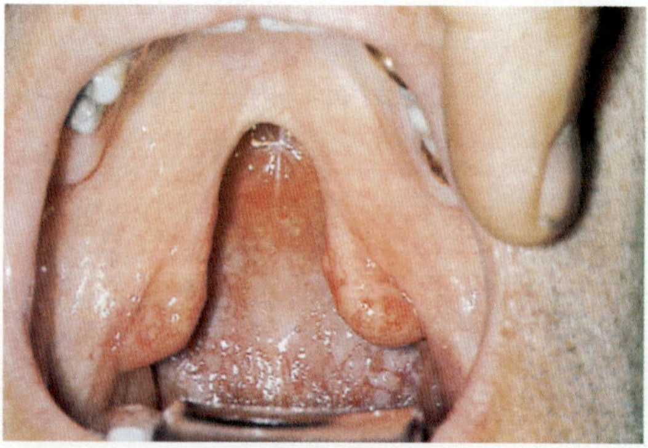

图 127　成人未经治疗的腭裂
Untreated cleft palate in an adult.

喉的临床检查

若声嘶、吞咽困难、慢性咽痛或持续性颈部包块超过六周，则必须行仔细的上呼吸道检查。聆听患者的声音，看是间断性还是持续性发音困难。前者可能是功能性的病变，而后者则可能是器质性的病变。呼气音是声带麻痹的典型表现。同时，聆听是否有喉喘鸣，似口内含物音则提示声门上或口咽部病变。

评估口腔、口咽部时，需特别注意黏膜溃疡和肿胀性病变。若咽反射敏感，硬腭及口咽部应予以利多卡因表面麻醉以行间接喉镜检查。当医生轻持住患者伸出的舌头时，可由温热喉镜观察其喉部（图 128）。患者需经口呼吸。当指示患者发“Hey”音时，可观察到声带的运动。若患者不能耐受此检查，可将其鼻腔局部麻醉后以纤维内镜观察喉及下咽（图 129）。

鼻部和颈部应视为上呼吸道常规检查的一部分。

38 Clinical examination of the larynx

If symptoms of hoarseness, dysphagia, chronic sore throat or a lump in the neck continue for longer than 6 weeks, careful examination of the upper airway is mandatory. Listen to the patient's voice: is it intermittently or permanently dysphonic? The former might suggest a functional problem, the latter an organic one. A 'breathy' voice is typical of a vocal cord palsy. Also, listen for evidence of stridor. A 'hot potato' voice is indicative of supraglottic or oropharyngeal pathology.

When assessing the oral cavity and oropharynx, particular attention should be paid to mucosal ulceration or swelling. If the patient has a particularly brisk gag reflex, the palate and oropharynx should be sprayed with Lidocaine prior to attempting indirect laryngoscopy. A warmed laryngeal mirror is used to visualize the larynx while the doctor gently holds the patient's protruded tongue (Fig. 128). The patient should mouth breathe. Vocal cord movement is assessed by asking the patient to say 'Hey!' If the technique is not tolerated, then the patient's better nasal airway is locally anaesthetized and a fibre-optic scope is used to examine the larynx and pharynx (Fig. 129).

Both the nose and neck should be routinely examined as part of the assessment of the upper airway.

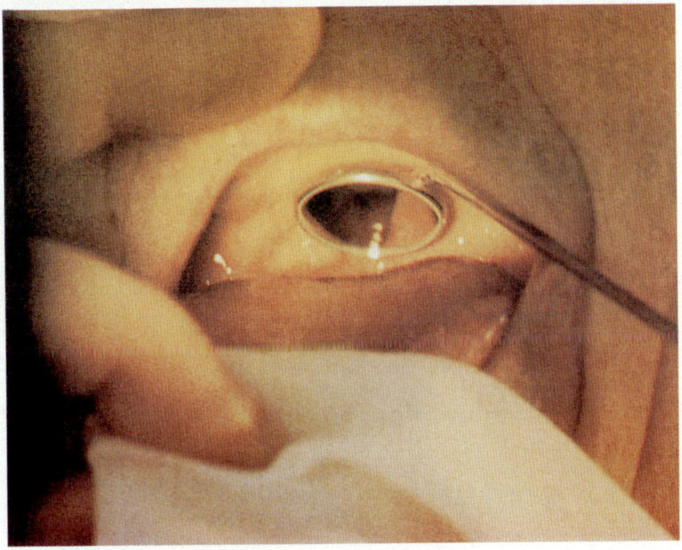

图 128　间接喉镜检查术
Indirect laryngoscopy.

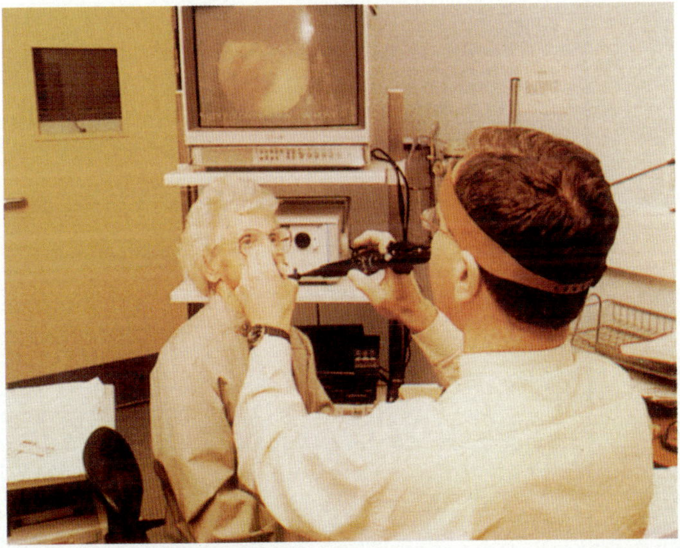

图 129　纤维喉镜检查术
Fibre-optic endoscopy.

39 慢性喉炎

慢性非特异性喉炎

病因

常由过度用声、吸烟或上呼吸道其他部位的化脓性感染引起，例如慢性鼻窦炎。

临床特征

声嘶，可伴有咽痛。间接喉镜检查可鉴别局限性病变和弥漫性病变，前者如声带小节（图130）、任克水肿（图131）或喉息肉，后者如慢性肥厚性喉炎（图132）。

治疗

治疗包括去除各种诱发因素和语音治疗。局限性息肉或小节可内镜下切除。

慢性特异性喉炎

少见。大部分的肉芽肿性疾病均可累及喉部，如：结核、梅毒、结节病、硬结病或韦格纳肉芽肿。

治疗

病损常似癌，直接喉镜检查和病理活检是必要的。以系统的全身治疗为主。

白斑

常累及真声带（图 133）。病因类似慢性非特异性喉炎。显微镜下通常可见过度角化和角化不全。需行活检以除外原位癌或侵袭性癌。

治疗

所有病例均应行内镜检查。白斑应视为癌前病变。

Chronic laryngitis

Chronic non-specific laryngitis

Aetiology

Common. Usually associated with vocal abuse, smoking or sepsis elsewhere in the respiratory tract, e.g. chronic sinusitis.

Clinical features

Hoarseness may be accompanied by sore throat. Indirect laryngoscopy may distinguish localized forms, e.g. singer's nodules (Fig. 130), Reinke's oedema (Fig. 131) or laryngeal polyps, from the generalized forms, e.g. chronic hypertrophic laryngitis (Fig. 132).

Management

Treatment involves the removal of any precipitating factors and speech therapy is important. Localized polyps or nodules may merit endoscopic removal.

Chronic specific laryngitis

Rare. Most of the granulomatous diseases can involve the larynx, e.g. tuberculosis, syphilis, sarcoidosis, scleroma or Wegener's granulomatosis.

Management

The lesions may mimic a carcinoma and a direct laryngoscopy and biopsy is mandatory. Treatment is that of the underlying systemic condition.

Leukoplakia

Usually affects the true cords (Fig. 133). The aetiology is as for chronic non-specific laryngitis. Microscopically, the findings of hyperkeratosis and dysplasia are common, although in situ or invasive carcinoma can only be excluded by an adequate biopsy.

Management

Endoscopy should be undertaken in all cases. Leukoplakia should be regarded as having the potential to undergo malignant change.

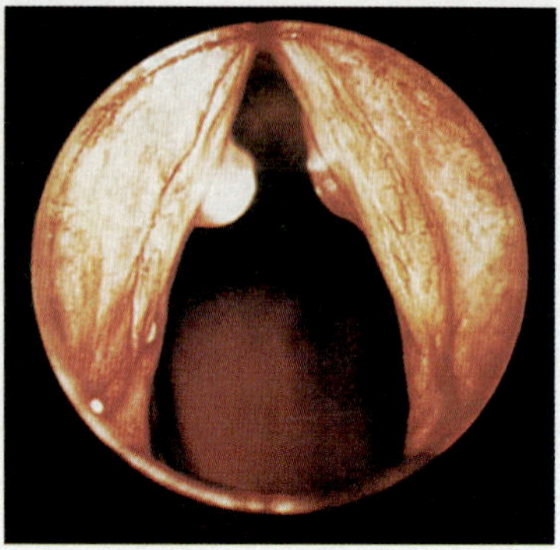

图 130　声带小节
Singer's nodules.

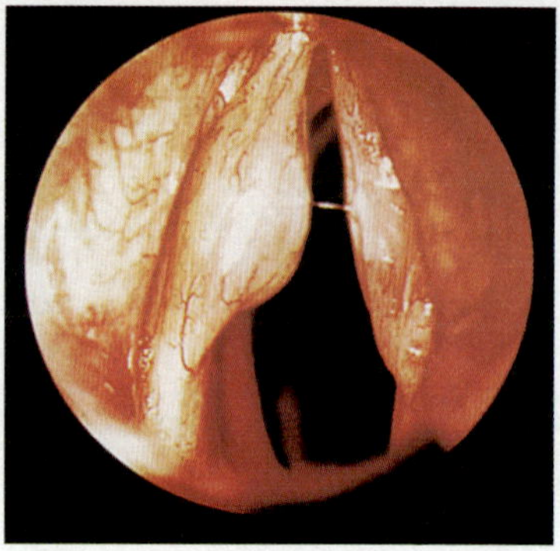

图 131　单侧任克水肿
Unilateral Reinke's oedema.

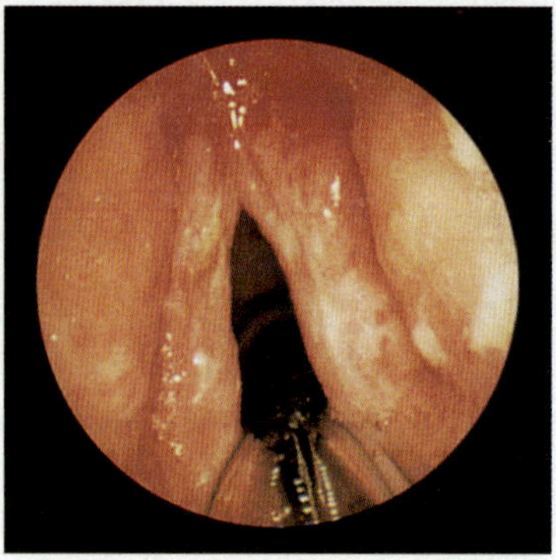

图 132　慢性肥厚性喉炎
Chronic hypertrophic laryngitis.

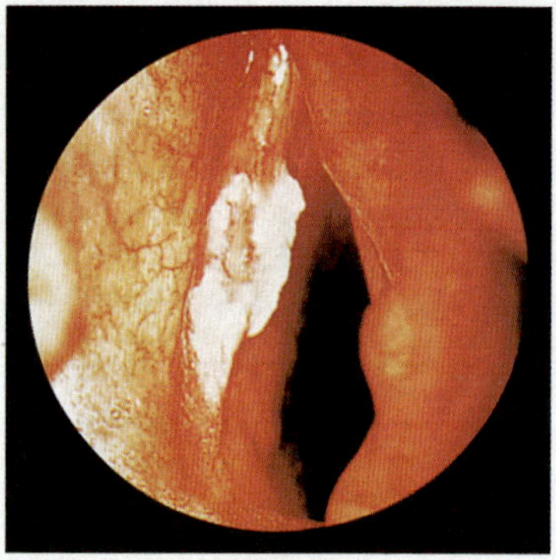

图 133　左声带白斑
Leukoplakia of the left true vocal cord.

乳头状瘤

病因 局部感染人乳头状瘤病毒（HPV）。

临床特征 在儿童（小儿型），多发性病损可扩展到气管、支气管。青春期肿瘤可消退。

在成人少见且多为单发。

均可表现为声嘶或呼吸道梗阻。

治疗 应用抽吸电热疗法或CO_2激光行内镜下切除（图 134）。喉及气管内的手术种植多见，术后易复发，因此常需多次手术治疗。

癌

病因 与吸烟和大量饮酒相关，而后者多引起梨状窝癌。

临床特征 通常表现为持续性声嘶。亦可出现吞咽困难、慢性咳嗽、喉喘鸣和反射性耳痛。声门上型喉癌有时伴有颈淋巴结转移。间接喉镜可以观察到肿瘤，但在明确治疗方案前应行内镜下评估（图 135）和病理活检。需排除上呼吸消化道的多重癌（1%）的发生。可疑颈部包块的细针抽吸活检亦为必要。CT扫描可显示肿瘤的喉外侵犯或喉软骨是否受累。

40 Laryngeal tumours

Papilloma

Aetiology

Localized infection with human papillomavirus (HPV).

Clinical features

In the child (juvenile form): multiple lesions that may spread to the trachea and bronchi. Cases may regress at puberty.

In the adult: less common and usually a single lesion.

Both forms present with hoarseness or airway obstruction.

Management

Endoscopic removal (Fig. 134) using either suction diathermy or a CO_2 laser. Surgical seeding of lesions within the larynx or trachea is common, and removal may be necessary for frequent recurrence.

Carcinoma

Aetiology

Associated with cigarette smoking and high alcohol intake, although the latter is more important in causing piriform fossa carcinoma.

Clinical features

Usually presents as persistent hoarseness. Dysphagia, chronic cough, stridor and referred otalgia may also occur. Occasionally a supraglottic tumour may present with metastatic neck nodes. The tumour may be evident on indirect laryngoscopy but endoscopic assessment (Fig. 135) and biopsy are mandatory before deciding on the appropriate treatment. A second primary (1%) in the upper aerodigestive tract should be searched for at this time.
Fine-needle aspiration cytology of any suspicious neck mass should also be undertaken. A CT scan will show any spread outside the larynx, or involvement of laryngeal cartilages.

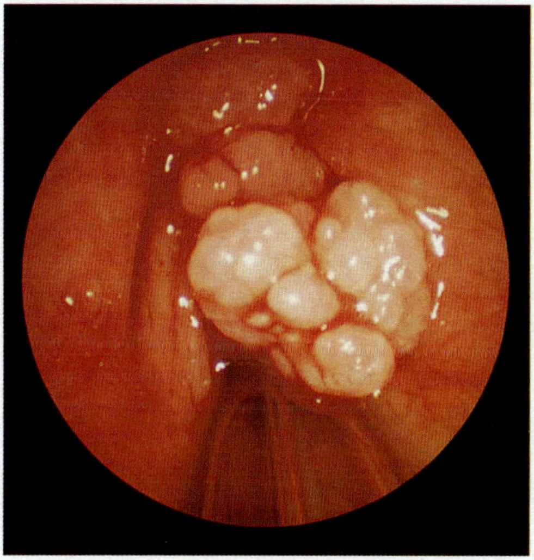

图 134　喉乳头状瘤的内镜下所见
Endoscopic appearance of laryngeal papillomata.

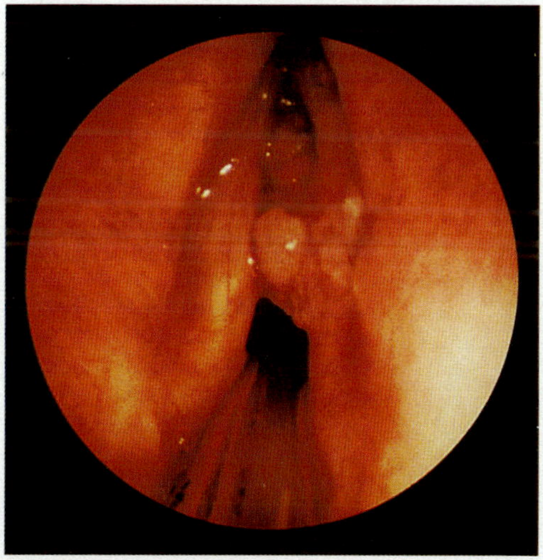

图 135　早期的右声带癌
Early right vocal cord carcinoma.

治疗

小的（T1和T2）病变可先行放疗，喉切除手术治疗放疗后复发的病例及大的（T3和T4）病变（图136）和伴有转移颈淋巴结直径大于2cm的病变。目前有些医师正在开展喉癌的内镜下CO_2激光切除术。

语音康复

全喉术后患者可通过以下途径发声：

1. 学习食管发音（吞咽空气然后主动通过食道入口自咽部流出）。
2. 应用人工喉（图138），当患者做构音动作时，其振动可被传导至咽和口腔。
3. 手术行气管食管造瘘，通过瘘口安装发音钮或活瓣（图137）。发音钮为单向活瓣，当气管造瘘口堵住时气流能由气管通向咽腔。部分病例可由此获得较高质量的发音。

结果

患者需密切随访。复发可发生于喉、咽、造瘘口或颈部。复发后可行手术或放疗。T1病例的5年生存率可达95%，而T4病例则降至50%。

Management

Small (T1 and T2) carcinomas are best treated with primary radiotherapy, laryngectomy being reserved for post-radiation recurrences, larger (T3 and T4) lesions (Fig. 136) and primary tumours associated with neck nodes greater than 2 cm in diameter. Primary endoscopic excision of laryngeal carcinomas with a carbon dioxide laser is now being undertaken by some surgeons.

Voice rehabilitation

Following total laryngectomy the patient may be able to speak again by:

- learning oesophageal speech (swallowed air is voluntarily regurgitated through the pharynx)
- using an artificial larynx (Fig. 138), which transmits vibrations into the pharynx and oral cavity while the patient articulates
- surgical provision of a tracheo-oesophageal fistula, which is fitted with a button or valve (Fig. 137). The button has a one-way flutter valve, which allows airflow from the trachea into the pharynx when the tracheostome is occluded. In selected patients this enables the development of good voice.

Results

Patients require close follow-up. Recurrences can develop in the larynx, pharynx, stoma or neck. Further surgery or radiotherapy may be indicated. The expected 5-year survival for a T1 laryngeal cancer is about 95%. This falls to about 50% for T4 disease.

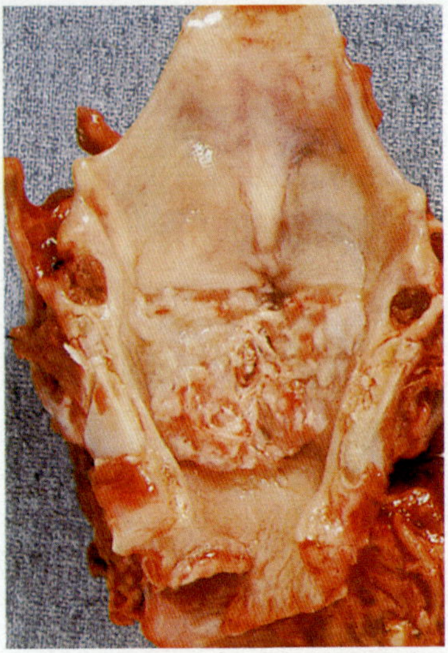

图 136 手术标本显示侵及范围广泛的喉癌
Operative specimen showing extensive laryngeal carcinoma.

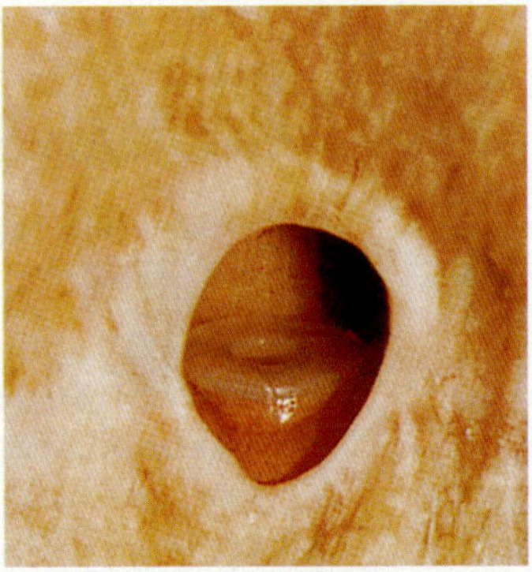

图 137 Blom-Singer 发音钮
Blom-Singer valve in situ.

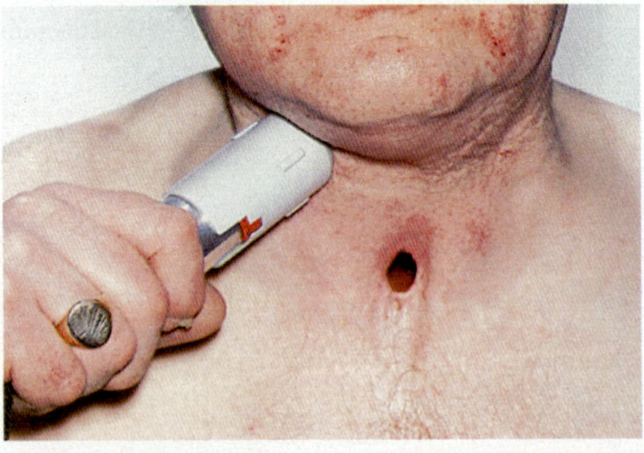

图 138 患者使用的人工喉
Patient using an 'artificial larynx'.

上呼吸消化道异物

口咽

鱼刺可扎在扁桃体或舌根。

临床特征 患者主诉吞咽痛，且多指向舌骨上区域。鱼刺有时需要触诊方能探及，X 线检查对于诊断没有帮助。

治疗 直视下取出鱼刺。

下咽 / 食管

骨头或球状食物常存留于以下四个部位：

一侧梨状隐窝
环后区（距上切牙 15cm）
主动脉弓水平（距上切牙 25cm）
食管胃结合处（距上切牙 40cm）

临床特征 完全性的吞咽困难，流涎且梗阻感指向胸骨上区或胸骨后区。颈部侧位软组织 X 线片可能显示骨头的轮廓（图 139）。

治疗 尽快行内镜下异物取出，以防呼吸道水肿、软组织感染或食管穿孔。

支气管

支气管异物常为坚果类食物，多发生于小儿。

临床特征 在最初的呛咳后呼吸窘迫出现前通常有一段隐匿期。若梗阻是完全的，则 X 线可示异物远端的肺部塌陷。若梗阻局部形成单向通气活瓣，则可导致患侧肺气肿（图 140）。

治疗 支气管镜下异物取出。

41 Upper aerodigestive tract foreign bodies

Oropharynx

Fish bones may lodge in the tonsil or tongue base.

Clinical features

The patient complains of pain on swallowing and points to the suprahyoid region. The bone may only be obvious on palpation: X-rays are unhelpful.

Management

Removal under direct vision.

Hypopharynx/oesophagus

A bone or food bolus usually gets lodged at one of four sites:

- one piriform fossa
- the postcricoid region (15cm from the upper incisor)
- the level of the aortic arch (at 25cm)
- at the oesophago-gastric junction (40cm).

Clinical features

Dysphagia may be total, the patient spitting out saliva and pointing to the suprasternal or retrosternal region. A soft tissue lateral X-ray of the neck may delineate a bone (Fig. 139).

Management

Endoscopic removal should be undertaken as soon as possible, to avoid airway oedema, soft tissue infection or oesophageal perforation.

Bronchus

Often a peanut in a young child.

Clinical features

After an initial coughing fit there is often a latent period before respiratory distress becomes obvious. The chest X-ray may show collapse of the lung distally, if the obstruction is complete, or emphysema of the involved side if the obstruction acts as a one-way valve (Fig. 140).

Management

Bronchoscopic removal is mandatory.

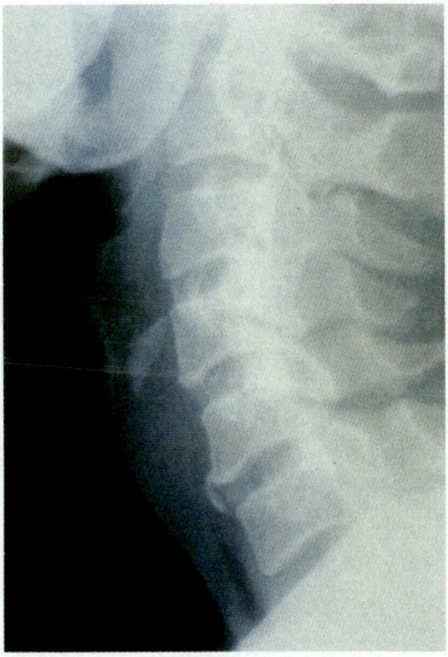

图 139　下咽腔内的鸡骨
Chicken bone in hypopharynx.

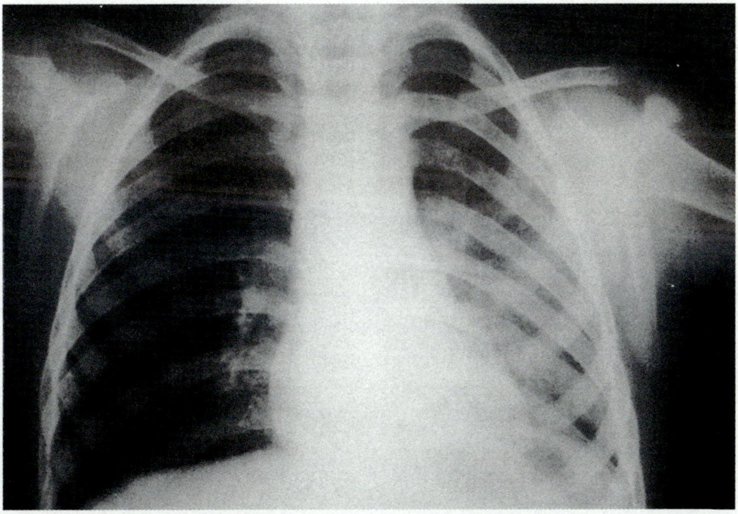

图 140　右主支气管腔内的坚果，可见同侧肺气肿
Peanut in right main bronchus, demonstrating ipsilateral emphysema.

先天性颈部肿块

甲状舌管囊肿

为颈中线最常见的囊肿（图 141），常在儿时发病。

临床特征 肿物可随伸舌动作而上下移动，继发感染可引起疼痛。窦道可继发于先前的感染或不彻底的切除手术。

治疗 行甲状腺功能扫描，若能在肿物范围以外发现有功能的甲状腺组织，则应将肿物行手术切除。应同时切除中份舌骨体并沿囊肿蒂追踪至舌盲孔一并切除（Sistrunk 手术）。

鳃裂囊肿及瘘管

病因 为胚胎时期鳃器的残余。第二鳃囊和颈窦退化不全可导致瘘管形成。

临床特征 囊肿常位于胸锁乳突肌前缘深面，表现为无痛性颈部肿胀；当继发感染时，其临床表现可类似于咽旁脓肿。完整的瘘管其内口位于扁桃体区，外口则位于胸锁乳突肌前缘。针吸囊肿内容物可以确诊。

治疗 手术切除，务必切净所有病变，包括瘘管各个分支。

水囊状淋巴管瘤

为淋巴管瘤的一种。

临床特征 通常为位于腮腺区的质软、透光肿物(图 142)，多在一岁以内发病。

治疗 手术切除。但常因肿瘤细胞弥漫浸润周围软组织而不易切净。

Congenital neck masses

Thyroglossal cyst

Most common midline neck cyst (Fig. 141) usually presenting in childhood.

Clinical features Painless, unless infected, and moves on protrusion of tongue. Sinus formation may follow previous infection or incomplete excision.

Management If a thyroid scan shows functioning tissue elsewhere, then excise with central portion of hyoid bone and tract up to foramen caecum (Sistrunk's operation).

Branchial cyst and fistula

Aetiology Represent branchial apparatus remnants. The fistula results from persistence of the second pouch and cervical sinus.

Clinical features Cysts usually lie deep to the anterior border of sternomastoid, presenting with a painless neck swelling or mimicking a parapharyngeal abscess if infection occurs. A complete branchial fistula has its internal opening in the region of the tonsil and an external opening anterior to sternomastoid. Diagnosis can be confirmed by needle aspiration of cyst contents.

Management Excision, with any fistulous tract.

Cystic hygroma

A variety of lymphangioma.

Clinical features A soft, transilluminable mass usually presenting in the parotid region in the first year of life (Fig. 142).

Management Excision, which may have to be incomplete because of the diffuse infiltration of soft tissues by the tumour.

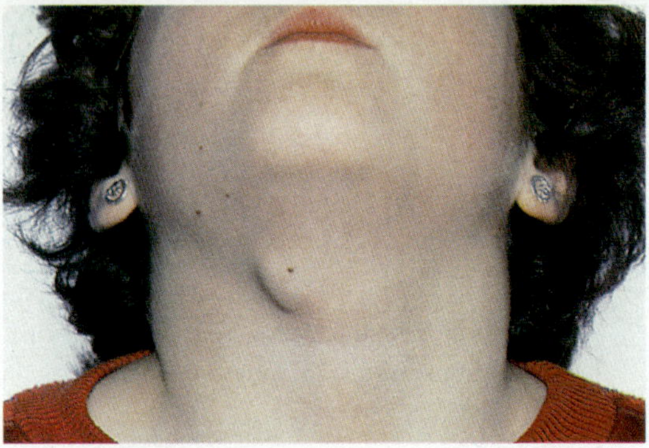

图 141　甲状舌管囊肿
Thyroglossal cyst.

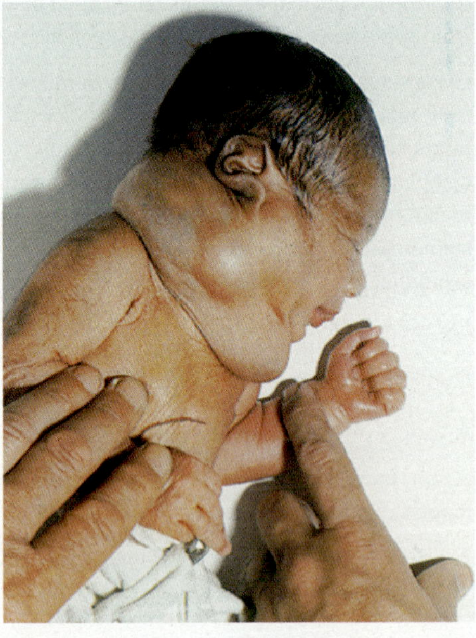

图 142　右腮腺水囊状淋巴管瘤
Cystic hygroma of the right parotid gland.

气管造口术

气管造口术即在气管前壁造口，使气管管腔经颈前与外界相通的手术。气管造瘘可为永久性，如喉全切除术后；在保留喉功能的前提下，亦可行暂时性气管切开（图 143）。

适应证

- 喉全切除术；
- 保持气道通畅，如在头颈部大手术后，或神经性疾病使喉功能受累时；
- 气道阻塞性疾病，如急性会厌炎、双侧喉返神经麻痹和肿瘤等；
- 呼吸功能障碍（气管插管时间需要超过 72 小时），如严重胸廓外伤、格林 - 巴利综合征等。

手术技巧

- 切口：在环状软骨与胸骨上切迹连线中点水平作横切口。
- 沿颈白线纵行切开并向两侧分离带状肌。
- 切断和分离甲状腺峡部。
- 行气管切开。在成人应行气管前壁开窗（图 144），在儿童则只作一纵行切口。切忌行活瓣形造口。
- 置入适当管径的气管套管。在头 24 小时内，可使用带气囊的气管套管；24 小时后可改为不带气囊的套管。

43 Tracheostomy

A tracheostomy is an artificial opening made into the trachea. It may be created after the larynx has been removed, when it is permanent, or when the larynx is still in place, when it is usually temporary (Fig. 143).

Indications

- Total laryngectomy
- Airway protection, e.g. after major head and neck surgery, neurological disease involving the larynx
- Airway obstruction, e.g. epiglottitis, bilateral recurrent laryngeal nerve palsy, tumour
- Respiratory insufficiency (when endotracheal intubation required for longer than 72h), e.g. severe chest wall injury, Guillain-Barré syndrome.

Surgical technique

- Incision. Horizontal, midway between the cricoid cartilage and suprasternal notch.
- Vertical incision and separation of strap muscles.
- Transfixion and separation of thyroid isthmus.
- Creation of an opening into the trachea. In adults a window is cut out (Fig. 144). A vertical slit incision is used in children. A trap-door flap should not be used.
- Insertion of tracheostomy tube. A correctly sized cuffed synthetic tube is used for the first 24 h. This can be replaced later on by an uncuffed tube (Fig. 145).

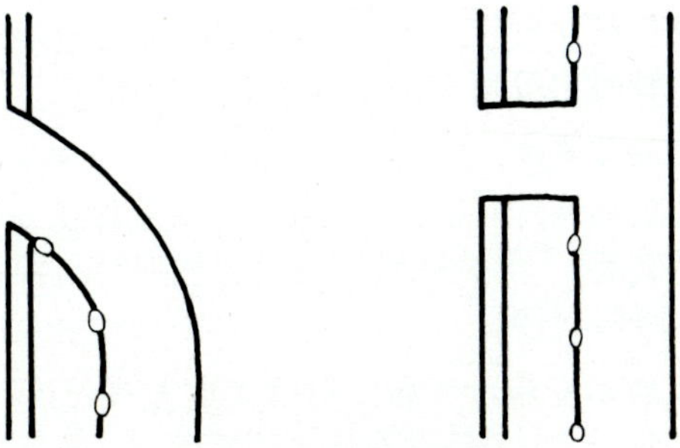

图 143　不同类型的气管造口术
Types of tracheostomy.

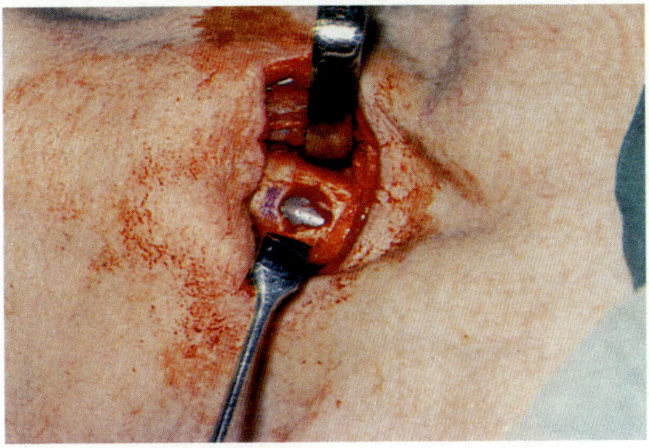

图 144　气管前壁开窗
Window cut in anterior tracheal wall.

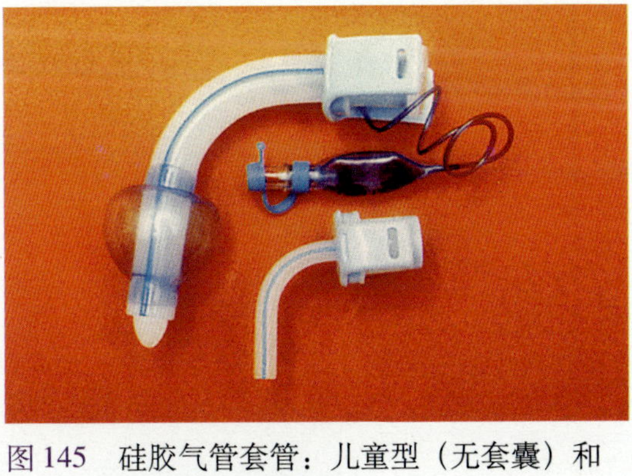

图 145　硅胶气管套管：儿童型（无套囊）和成人型（带套囊）
Silicone tracheostomy tubes: paediatric uncuffed and adult cuffed.

手术并发症

急性期并发症：气胸、大出血、术后皮下气肿及气管插管脱出等可在术中或术后立即出现。

早期并发症：常见的有切口感染、吞咽困难和气管插管阻塞等。罕见的并发症有气管壁坏死（可伴无名动脉破裂）、气管软骨膜炎及通气突然改善引起的反射性呼吸暂停。

晚期并发症：气囊压迫过久或充气过度可导致气管狭窄。这可导致儿童患者拔管困难。拔管后气管造瘘口一般无需进行手术缝合，多可自行封闭。

造瘘口狭窄

病因

喉全切除术后，气管下端与造瘘口周围皮肤缝合。局部伤口感染、放疗及瘢痕形成等均易导致造瘘口狭窄（图 146）。另外，肿瘤复发亦可造成造瘘口狭窄（图 147）。

治疗

良性造瘘口狭窄患者可永久配戴造瘘口钮或气管套管或行手术扩大造瘘口。

Complications

Immediate. Pneumothorax, haemorrhage, surgical emphysema and tube displacement can all occur.

Early. Wound infection, dysphagia and tube obstruction are all common. Tracheal erosion with innominate artery rupture, perichondritis and apnoea in hypercapnoeic bronchitics are rare.

Late. Tracheal stenosis may result from prolonged or overinflation of the cuffed tube. Decannulation may be difficult in children. Surgical closure of a persistent tracheocutaneous fistula is rarely required after decannulation.

Stomal stenosis

Aetiology

Following laryngectomy the lower end of the trachea is brought out through the neck skin. Local wound infection, radiotherapy and keloid formation all predispose to the later development of a stomal stenosis (Fig. 146). The other cause of stomal stenosis is recurrence of tumour (Fig. 147).

Management

Management of benign stomal stenosis is either by the permanent wearing of a stoma button or laryngectomy tube or by surgical revision of the stoma.

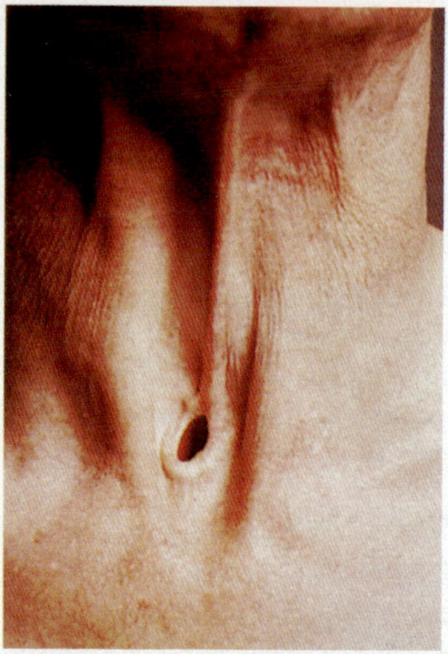

图 146　气管造瘘口瘢痕性狭窄
Stomal stenosis due to scar tissue.

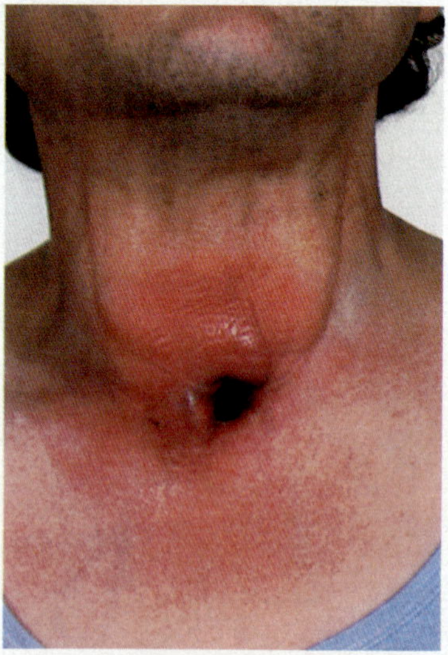

图 147　喉癌喉全切除术后气管造瘘口复发
Post-laryngectomy stomal recurrence.

喉部及咽部憩室

咽囊

病因 咽囊系由下咽部黏膜经 Killian 裂孔疝出而形成的。

临床特征 吞咽困难及食物反流为其临床表现。巨大的咽囊还可引起吸入性肺炎。间接喉镜下可见下咽腔内唾液潴留。上述临床症状结合钡餐造影可明确诊断（图 148）。

治疗 首先经内镜检查排除肿瘤可能。可经颈外入路切除囊袋，亦可用枪形吻合器在内镜下切除病变，咽管断端可直接吻合（图 149）。

喉膨出

病因 喉黏膜囊性扩张即形成内生性或外生性喉膨出（图 150）。

临床特征 最常见的有声嘶和吞咽困难。形成颈部包块者在做 Valsalva动作时，包块可明显增大。在做Valsalva动作同时行喉部断层扫描可清楚显示喉膨出（图 151）。

治疗 内镜下除外肿瘤。内生性膨出可经内镜直接完整囊外切除，外生性膨出须经颈外入路切除。

44 Diverticula of the larynx and pharynx

Pharyngeal pouch

Aetiology

A pharyngeal pouch develops from a herniation of pharyngeal mucosa through Killian's dehiscence.

Clinical features

Dysphagia and regurgitation of food occur. Large pouches may cause aspiration pneumonia. Pooling of saliva in the hypopharynx may be noted on indirect laryngoscopy. Barium swallow confirms the diagnosis (Fig. 148).

Management

Following an endoscopy to exclude an associated carcinoma, the pouch may be excised via an external approach or the wall between the pouch and oesophagus divided endoscopically using a stapling gun (Fig. 149).

Laryngocele

Aetiology

Distension of the laryngeal saccule can produce an internal or external laryngocele (Fig. 150).

Clinical features

Hoarseness or dysphagia may occur. External laryngoceles may produce a swelling in the neck accentuated by performing Valsalva's manoeuvre. Laryngeal tomograms taken during this manoeuvre will demonstrate the laryngocele (Fig. 151).

Management

Following endoscopy to exclude an associated carcinoma, an internal laryngocele can be 'uncapped' whilst an external laryngocele is excised through the neck.

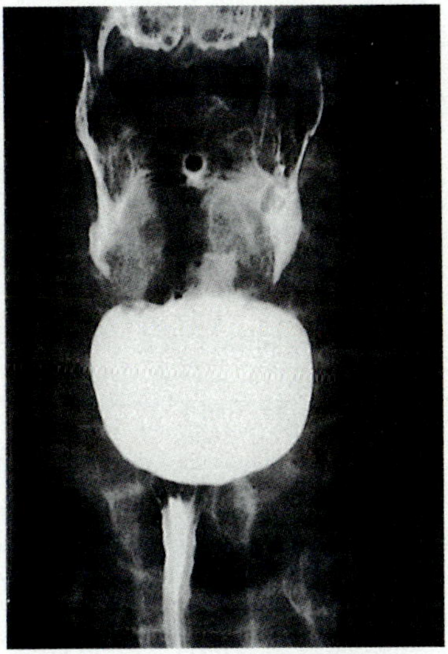

图 148　钡餐造影显示咽囊
Barium swallow demonstrating a pharyngeal pouch.

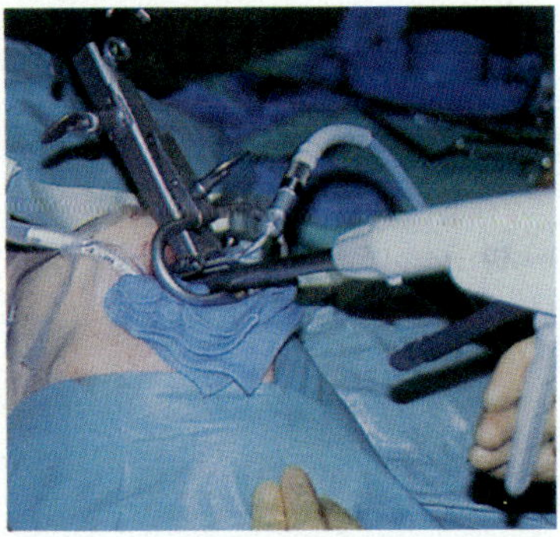

图 149　内镜下使用枪形吻合器治疗咽囊
The use of an endoscopic stapling gun for the treatment of a pharyngeal pouch.

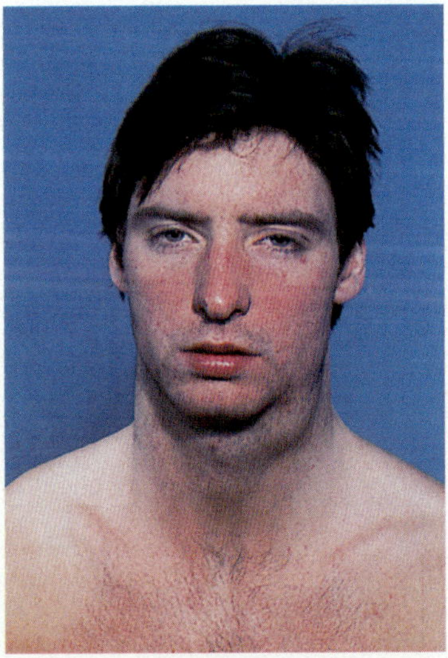

图 150　外生性喉膨出患者颈部包块
Patient with an external laryngocele.

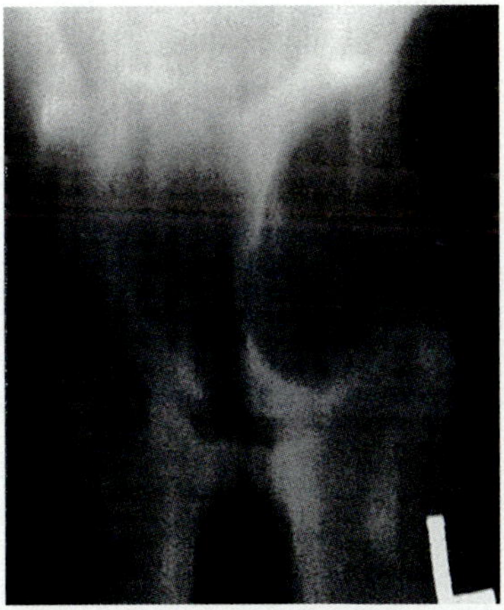

图 151　X 线体层摄影显示含气的喉膨出
Tomogram outlining air-filled laryngocele.

45 口底疾病

口底解剖

口底主要由舌前2/3和舌两侧黏膜向下颌牙龈反折所构成。在口底，双侧下颌下腺导管开口于舌下阜，由位于中线的舌系带将其分隔开，左右各一。舌下腺位于口底黏膜下。

舌下囊肿（Ranula 囊肿）

病因

为起源于舌下腺的囊性病变。通常表现为口底发蓝、有波动感的肿物（图 152）。有时 Ranula 囊肿可表现为颈部肿块，称“跃进型 Ranula 囊肿”，较少见。

治疗

对于局限于口底的病变，可行袋形缝合治疗，但可能复发。跃进型囊肿则需经颈外入路完整切除。

鳞状细胞癌

临床特征

可表现为口底痛性溃疡，并伴有耳部反射痛（图 153）。早期颈淋巴结转移多见，可为双侧。

治疗

手术切除并行整形外科修复，再辅以局部放疗。

Diseases of the floor of the mouth

Anatomy

Formed largely by the anterior two-thirds of the tongue and by reflection of mucosa from the sides of the tongue to the gum on the mandible. In the midline the lingual frenulum separates the orifices of the left and right submandibular ducts. Under the mucosa lie the sublingual salivary glands.

Ranula

Aetiology A cystic lesion arising from the sublingual gland. Usually presents in the floor of the mouth as a bluish, fluctuant swelling (Fig. 152). Less commonly the 'plunging ranula' can present as a lump in the neck.

Treatment For lesions confined to the floor of the mouth, marsupialization is usually adequate, although recurrence can occur. Plunging ranulae require formal excision via an external neck approach.

Squamous carcinoma

Clinical features An ulcer in the floor of the mouth which may be painful with referred otalgia (Fig. 153). Early spread to cervical nodes, which may be bilateral, is common.

Treatment Excision of the tumour with plastic surgical reconstruction and adjuvant radiotherapy.

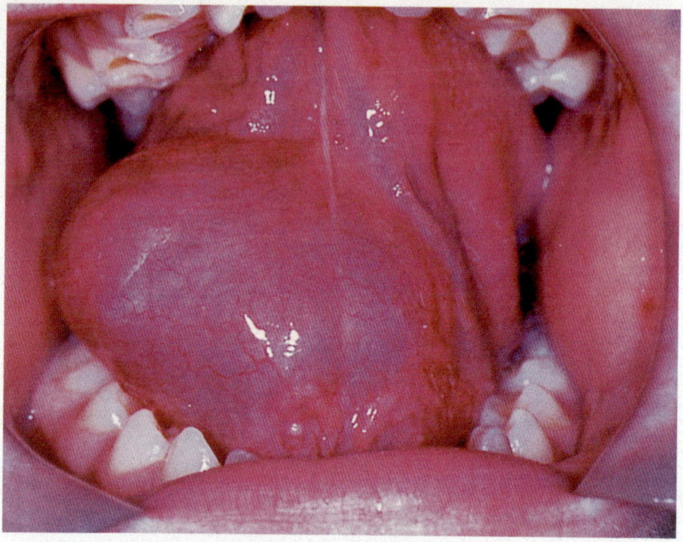

图 152　口底 Ranula 囊肿（舌下囊肿）
Ranula of the floor of the mouth.

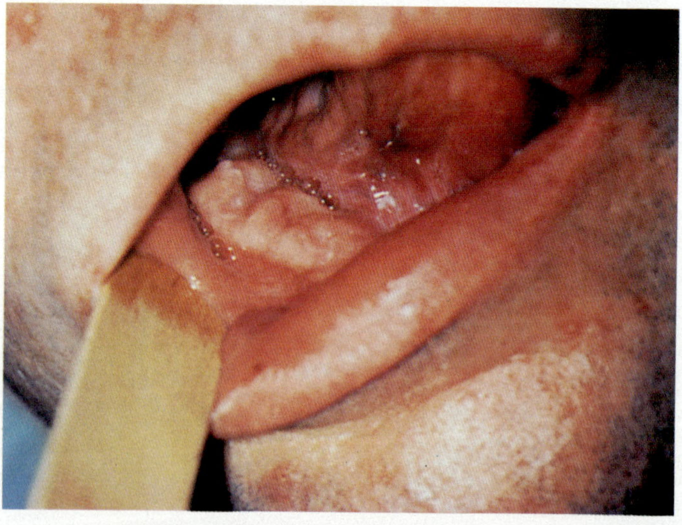

图 153　口底癌
Carcinoma of the floor of the mouth.

下颌下腺疾病

下颌下腺被下颌舌骨肌分为浅、深两部：浅部位于该肌浅面，深部则绕该肌后缘进入口底。下颌下腺导管（Wharton 管）自腺体的深部发出，前行并于中线旁舌下阜开口于口底。

感染或肿瘤等因素均可导致下颌下腺肿胀（图 154）。

炎症

临床特征

腺体肿胀、触痛常提示导管内结石。双合诊可触及，亦可在X线平片上显影（图 155）。颌下三角内有少量淋巴结，因此，当这些淋巴结肿大时易与下颌下腺疾病混淆。

治疗

应用抗生素及经口摘除结石。如果口内途径摘除结石有困难，可经颈外入路行下颌下腺摘除。此外，感染亦可导致脓肿形成。

肿瘤

疑及肿瘤者应行细针抽吸活检。下颌下腺肿瘤大约 50% 为良性，其中以多形性腺瘤最多见。

治疗

将肿瘤与下颌下腺一并切除，术中应注意保护面神经下颌缘支。对某些恶性肿瘤，还应同时行根治性颈清扫术。

46 Diseases of the submandibular gland

The superficial portion of the gland lies on the mylohyoid muscle; the deep portion extends around the posterior edge of muscle into the floor of the mouth. Wharton's duct leaves the deep part of the gland and runs forward to open into the anterior floor of the mouth, just lateral to the midline.

Swelling of the gland may be due to inflammation or tumour (Fig. 154).

Inflammatory disease

Clinical features

A tense, tender swelling usually results from a stone in the duct. This may be palpable bi-manually or evident on X-ray (Fig. 155). There are several lymph nodes in the submandibular triangle and enlargement of these may mimic disease in the gland.

Management

Treatment is with antibiotics and excision of the stone perorally. If this cannot be achieved, the whole gland may need to be removed by an external approach. Established infection may proceed to abscess formation.

Tumours

Fine-needle aspiration of the mass should be performed. About 50% of tumours are benign, most commonly pleomorphic adenomas.

Management

These should be excised with the entire gland, taking care to preserve the marginal mandibular branch of the facial nerve. Malignant tumours necessitate excision of the whole gland, with a radical neck dissection in certain cases.

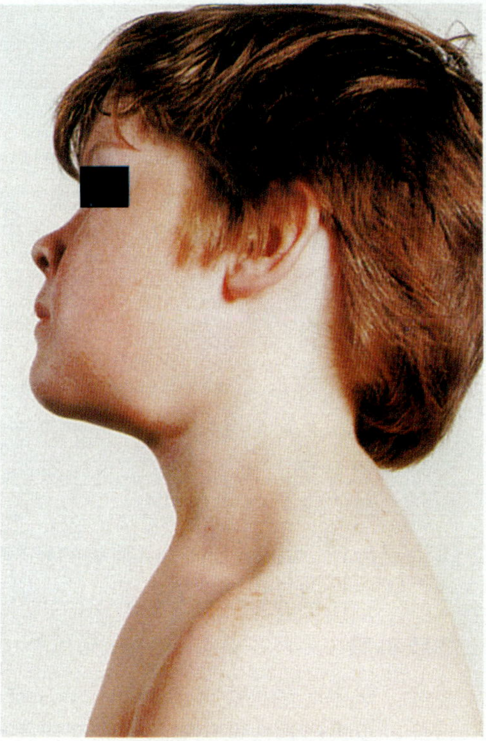

图 154　慢性感染导致下颌下腺肿大
Enlargement of the submandibular gland due to chronic infection.

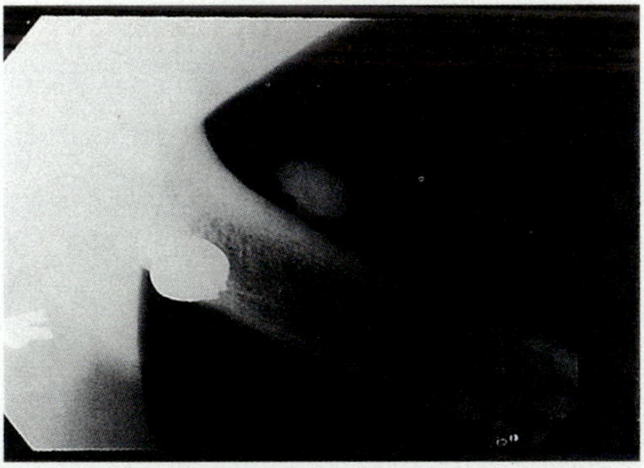

图 155　口底 X 线片显示下颌下腺导管结石
Floor of mouth X-ray demonstrating a stone in the submandibular gland duct.

腮腺膨大性疾病

流行性腮腺炎

临床特征 本病由腮腺炎病毒引起，常见于儿童，是引起双侧腮腺肿大的最常见原因（图 156）。临床表现为双侧腮腺区疼痛及触痛。

治疗 支持治疗。腮腺肿胀可在治疗数日后消退。

急性腮腺脓肿

常见于口腔卫生不良的患者，伴或不伴龋齿。

临床特征 腮腺明显触痛，局部有明显的软组织炎症表现（图 157）。触诊或 X 线平片可发现导管内结石。

治疗 抗生素治疗，如治疗过程中肿胀的腮腺出现触诊波动感，则应当进行切开引流。手术径路同腮腺切除术。

腮腺肿瘤

分类 *良性*：如多形性腺瘤（图 158）、Warthin 瘤；
恶性：如腺样囊性癌、鳞状细胞癌或腺癌、淋巴瘤等。

临床特征 肿瘤通常呈无痛性，但快速增长者恶性可能性大。若有面瘫则高度提示恶性肿瘤。细针抽吸活检可帮助术前确诊。

治疗 对良性肿瘤只要求行腮腺浅叶切除。而对恶性肿瘤则须行腮腺全切术，并且同时切除面神经。

Parotid gland swellings

Mumps

Clinical features

Usually seen in children, this is the most common cause of bilateral parotid gland swelling (Fig.156). The glands are painful and tender.

Management

Treatment is supportive, the adenopathy subsiding over a period of several days.

Acute parotid abscess

Usually seen in association with poor oral hygiene, with or without dental caries.

Clinical features

The gland becomes acutely tender with obvious inflammation of the soft tissues (Fig. 157). A stone may be palpable in the duct or evident on plain X-ray.

Management

Treatment with antibiotics should be followed by drainage via a parotidectomy approach if the swelling becomes fluctuant.

Parotid gland tumours

Types

Benign: e.g. pleomorphic adenoma (Fig. 158), Warthin's tumour
Malignant: e.g. adenoid cystic, squamous cell or adenocarcinoma, lymphoma

Clinical features

Usually painless, the speed of growth reflects the likelihood of malignancy. A facial palsy indicates a malignant tumour. Fine-needle aspiration of the mass may facilitate preoperative diagnosis.

Management

Superficial parotidectomy should be undertaken when indicated. Malignant tumours may require a total parotidectomy with sacrifice of the facial nerve.

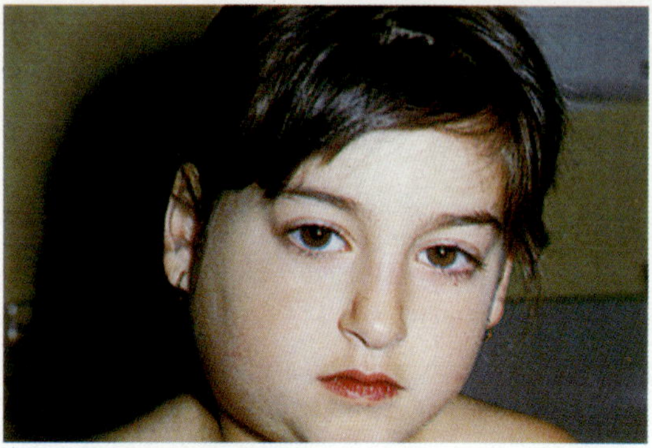

图 156　流行性腮腺炎
Mumps parotitis.

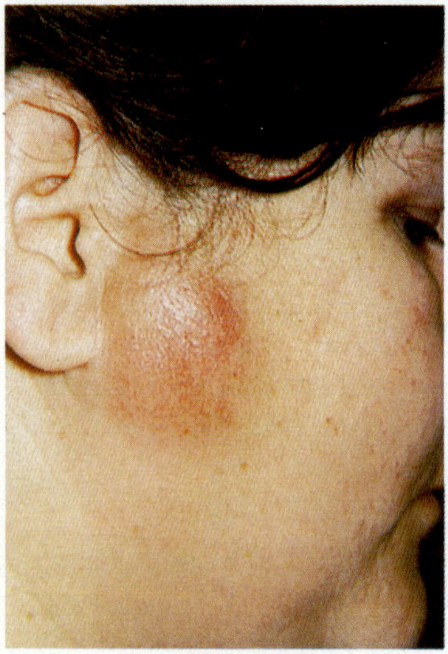

图 157　急性腮腺脓肿
Acute parotid abscess.

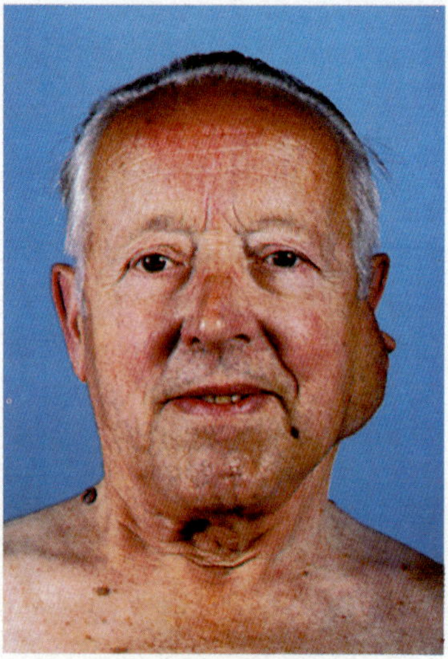

图 158　腮腺多形性腺瘤
Pleomorphic adenoma of the parotid gland.

头颈部缺损的手术修复 48

头颈部肿瘤切除术后的组织缺损，常因无法满足功能恢复或美观的要求而无法直接进行一期关闭。此时，要想获得满意的手术效果，就只能将身体其他部位的组织转移到术区，即进行修复手术。根据需要，供体组织既可用于黏膜缺损的修复，也可用于皮肤缺损的修复。

供体类型

无自带血供游离组织片：此种组织片无自带血供，须依靠受区血供方能存活，包括游离皮片、全厚皮片、真皮片、游离神经和骨组织等。

带蒂皮瓣：其血供可为随意性（指并非由某一条具体血管供血），或为轴型（由一条经解剖学命名的血管供血），如胸三角肌皮瓣（图 159）和胸大肌皮瓣（图 160）。

重建血供游离组织瓣：此种组织瓣本身带有供应血管，但需将其与受区血管重新吻合方能使组织瓣重新获得血供而存活。例如前臂游离皮瓣（图 161）和游离空肠等。

带蒂内脏：可取自胃、结肠等。

手术中应根据实际情况来决定供体组织的选择。

肌皮瓣和重建血供游离组织瓣可对腔面缺损行一期修复，从而大大缩短了住院时间。

48 Reconstruction in head and neck surgery

Following excision of a tumour from the head or neck, primary closure of a resultant tissue defect with preservation of adequate function may not be feasible or cosmetically acceptable. Only by the introduction of tissue from another site can a satisfactory result be achieved. Such tissue may be used to provide lining (reconstruction of an internal mucosal defect) or cover (reconstruction of a skin defect).

Techniques

Non-vascularized free grafts. These depend on the recipient site for their blood supply: include split skin, full-thickness skin, dermis, nerve and bone grafts.

Pedicled skin. May be random, with a non-specific blood supply, or axial, when the flap has a named arterial blood supply, e.g. deltopectoral flap (Fig. 159) and pectoralis major myocutaneous flap (Fig. 160).

Revascularized free grafts. The artery and vein supplying the graft tissue are re-anastomosed to vessels at the recipient site. Include radial forearm flap (Fig. 161) and jejunum.

Pedicled viscera. Stomach or colon may be used.

Several factors will determine the choice of flap/ graft for the individual patient.

Myocutaneous flaps and revascularized free grafts have meant that the lining of an internal surface can be carried out as a one-stage procedure, greatly reducing hospitalization time.

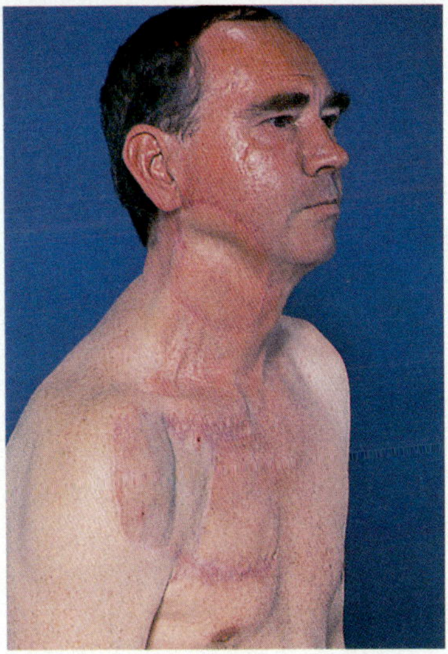

图 159　胸三角肌皮瓣修复颈部皮肤缺损
Neck skin replacement using a deltopectoral flap.

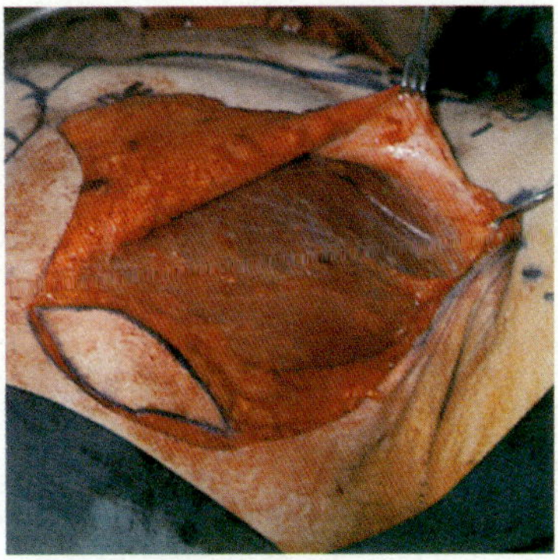

图 160　准备离断肌肉附着的胸大肌皮瓣
Pectoralis major flap just prior to division of the muscles' attachments.

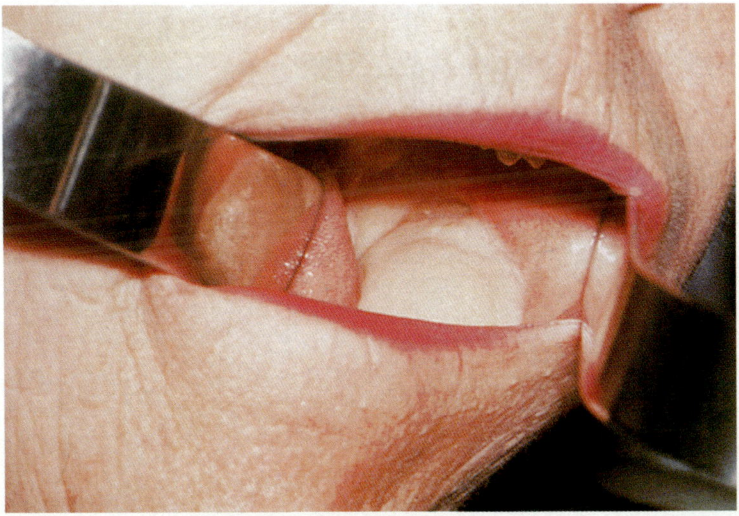

图 161　口腔内前臂游离皮瓣修复术后
Intra-orally placed radial free flap.

49 后四对脑神经麻痹

病因 常见于脑干或颅底病变，如心血管意外、运动神经元病、颈静脉球瘤、脑膜炎及鼻咽癌等。

舌咽神经（Ⅸ）麻痹

该神经支配咽黏膜及舌后1/3感觉（包括味觉），运动支支配咽中缩肌。

临床特征 该神经单独麻痹很少见，一侧麻痹多不影响整体功能。

迷走神经（Ⅹ）麻痹

该神经司喉部感觉及软腭、咽、喉的运动。同时还支配某些胸、腹内脏的感觉与运动。

病因 喉返神经为迷走神经的分支。单纯喉返神经麻痹常为特发性或由于该神经颈段或胸段损伤引起，如甲状腺切除术后或支气管癌等（图162）。

临床特征 迷走神经病变因发生部位的不同而表现各异。可出现软腭麻痹、声嘶、咳嗽无力、进食或咽喉分泌物呛咳、气道阻塞等。单纯喉返神经麻痹不会引起软腭麻痹。

治疗 一侧声带麻痹所致声门闭合不全可通过声门旁组织内注射聚四氟乙烯树脂以增大患侧声带体积来改善（图163）。可行甲状软骨成型术。双侧声带麻痹可导致气道完全阻塞或严重呛咳。此时可行气管造口术。

Palsies of the last four cranial nerves

Aetiology

Often involved with lesions in the brainstem or at the skull base, e.g. with CVA, motor neurone disease, glomus tumour, meningitis and nasopharyngeal carcinoma.

Glossopharyngeal nerve

This nerve is sensory to the posterior third of the tongue (including taste) and pharyngeal mucosa. Motor to middle constrictor.

Clinical features

It is rarely paralysed alone. A unilateral palsy does not produce severe functional disability.

Vagus nerve

This nerve is sensory to the larynx and motor to the soft palate, pharynx and larynx. Also sensorimotor to the thoraco-abdominal viscera.

Aetiology

An isolated palsy of the recurrent laryngeal branch is usually either idiopathic or due to disruption of the nerve in the neck or chest, e.g. post-thyroidectomy and bronchial carcinoma (Fig. 162).

Clinical features

Variable. Palatal paralysis, hoarseness, weak cough, overspill of food and secretions and airways obstruction may all occur, although a recurrent laryngeal nerve palsy will not produce palatal paralysis.

Management

Airway incompetence due to a unilateral cord palsy may be helped by injection of Teflon into the para-cordal tissues to increase the cord's bulk or a thyroplasty could be performed (Fig. 163). Bilateral palsies may produce total airway obstruction or serious overspill. A tracheostomy will be required in either case.

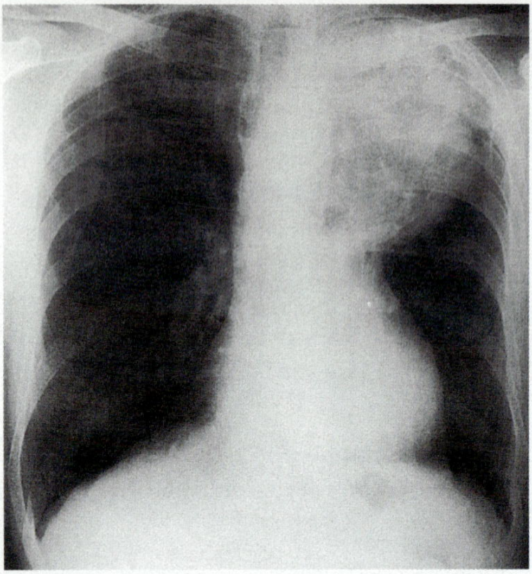

图 162 支气管肺癌导致左声带麻痹
Bronchial carcinoma causing a left vocal cord palsy.

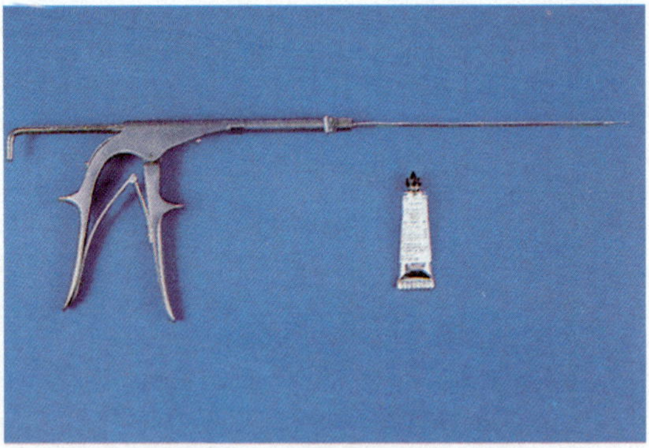

图 163 用于麻痹声带内镜注射的特氟隆枪
Teflon gun for endoscopic injection of a paralysed vocal cord.

副神经（XI）麻痹

该神经脊髓部支配胸锁乳突肌和斜方肌运动。单纯副神经麻痹常见于根治性颈廓清术后或不适当的V区淋巴结活检术。

临床特征 肩下垂（图 164），耸肩不能或肩部外展不能。

治疗 副神经损伤所致的凝肩通过理疗或可获益。

舌下神经（XII）麻痹

舌下神经支配舌体及舌骨下肌群的运动。单纯舌下神经麻痹常见于医源性损伤，如喉全切除术后或下颌下腺切除术后；亦可见于上颈部恶性肿瘤侵犯。

临床特征 伸舌时舌偏向患侧（图 165）。肌束震颤及萎缩提示下运动神经元损伤。单侧舌麻痹常无症状。双侧舌肌麻痹可导致严重的构音困难及吞咽困难。

Accessory nerve

The spinal part of this nerve is motor to sternomastoid and trapezius. An isolated palsy is seen after a block dissection of neck or injudicious posterior triangle lymph node biopsy.

Clinical features

The shoulder assumes a dropped appearance (Fig. 164) and the patient is unable to shrug or abduct the shoulder to a vertical position.

Management

A resultant frozen shoulder may benefit from physiotherapy.

Hypoglossal nerve

This nerve is motor to tongue and hyoid depressors. An isolated palsy is usually iatrogenic, e.g. following laryngectomy or submandibular gland excision, or due to malignant disease in the upper neck.

Clinical features

On protrusion the tongue deviates to the paralysed side (Fig. 165). Wasting and fasciculation indicate lower motor neurone damage. Unilateral palsies are usually asymptomatic. Bilateral palsies produce severe dysarthria and swallowing difficulties.

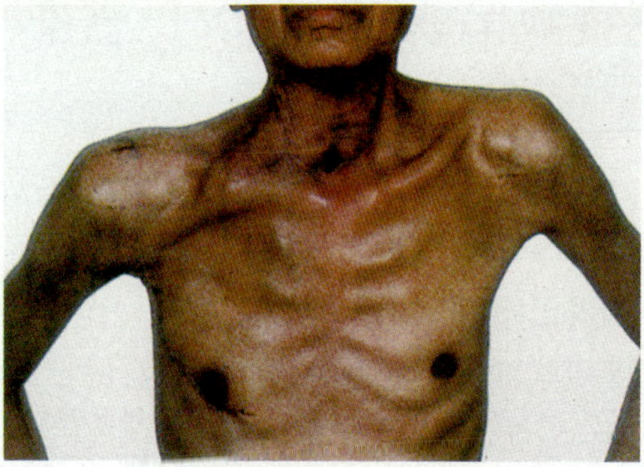

图 164　右颈廓清术（和喉切除术）后肩下垂
Dropped shoulder following right neck dissection (and laryngectomy).

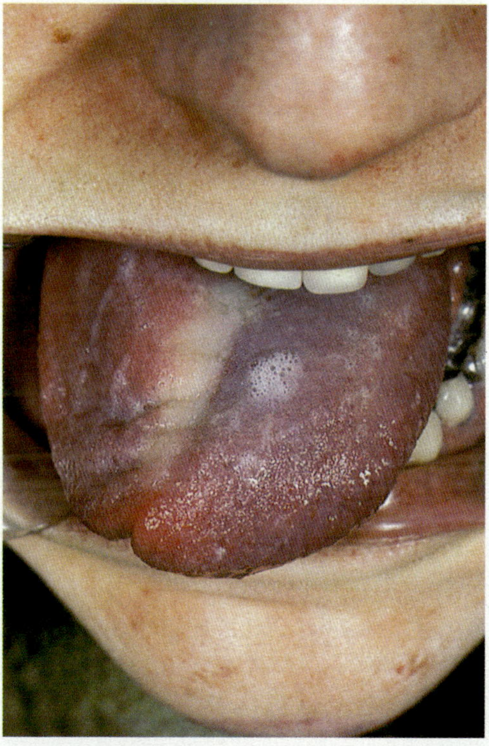

图 165　右舌下神经麻痹，伸舌时舌右偏，右侧舌肌萎缩
Hypoglossal nerve palsy with deviation and wasting of hemitongue.

50 人类免疫缺陷病毒（HIV）感染

在耳鼻咽喉科，人类免疫缺陷病毒感染常引起三大表现：

颈淋巴结肿大

临床特征 此症状常见。可能是持续性全身淋巴结肿大的一部分，也可能继发于咽炎。但是，快速增大、非对称性的（图 166）或固定的淋巴结则可能预示着淋巴瘤、Kaposi 肉瘤或隐匿性鳞状细胞癌的发生。

治疗 对于不能排除恶性肿瘤的病例，应当进行细针穿刺或开放活检，然后根据病理学结果来制定治疗计划。

Kaposi 肉瘤

Kaposi 肉瘤常常发生于艾滋病患者头颈部的皮肤和黏膜。

临床特征 病变表现为红色或紫色的斑疹、斑片或结节。腭部是最常见的受累部位（图 167）。极少数情况下，Kaposi 肉瘤也会引起气道阻塞。

治疗 综合治疗。

口腔毛状白斑

临床特征 口腔侧壁以及舌腹侧的白斑样斑块（图 168），可自行消退，也容易复发。该病损可能由 Epstein-Barr 病毒（EBV）感染导致。显微镜下可观察到螺旋状排列的角蛋白，形似毛发。该病须与艾滋病患者的另一种常见病损——念珠菌病鉴别。毛状白斑的出现往往预示着患者将很快进入艾滋病快速进展期。

治疗 活检确诊后应对病变进行临床观察。至于该病是否具有恶变倾向，目前尚未得知。

Human immunodeficiency virus (HIV) infection 50

ENT manifestations of HIV infection commonly fall into one of three groups.

Cervical lymphadenopathy

Clinical features

Common. May be persistent generalized lymphadenopathy (PGL) or secondary to pharyngitis. However, rapidly enlarging, asymmetrical (Fig. 166) or fixed nodes may herald a lymphoma, Kaposi's sarcoma or an occult squamous carcinoma.

Management

In cases where malignancy requires exclusion, fine-needle or open biopsy is necessary. The treatment will then depend on the pathological diagnosis.

Kaposi's sarcoma (KS)

The skin and mucosa of the head and neck are common sites for KS in AIDS patients.

Clinical features

Lesions present as red or purple macules, plaques or nodules. Palatal involvement is most common (Fig. 167). Rarely, KS may cause airway obstruction.

Management

Treatment is multi-modal.

Oral cavity 'hairy' leukoplakia

Clinical features

Leukoplakic patches on the lateral border and ventral surface of the tongue (Fig. 168) that have a tendency to regress and recur. Possibly caused by the Epstein-Barr virus (EBV). Microscopically the keratin whorls give a hairy appearance. The lesion should be distinguished from candidiasis, also common in these patients. Rapid progression to full blown AIDS is common once 'hairy' leukoplakia has developed.

Management

Treatment is by biopsy and observation of the lesion, the malignant potential of which remains unknown.

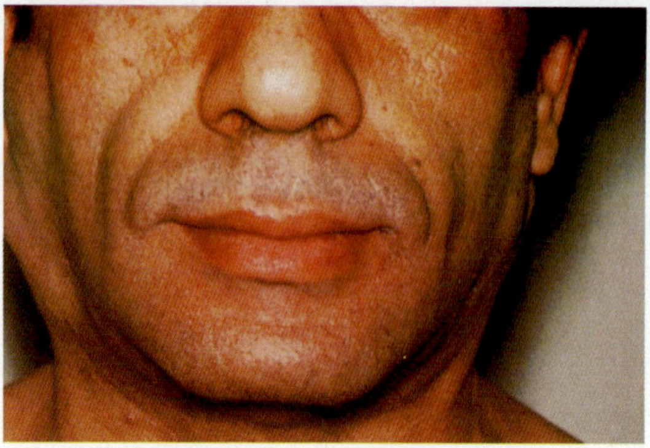

图 166　持续性全身淋巴结肿大患者非对称性颈淋巴结肿大
Asymmetrical cervical lymphadenopathy in PGL.

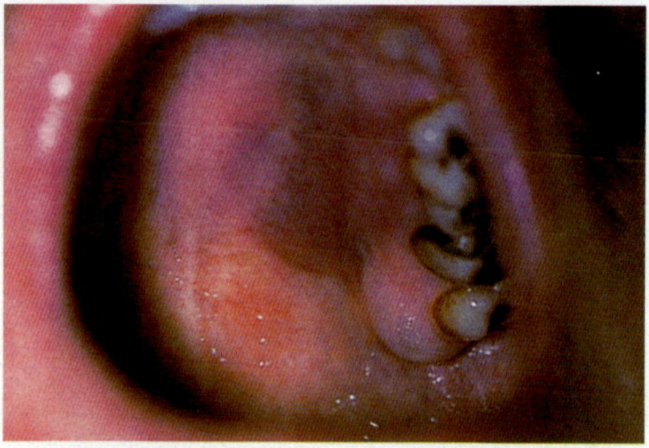

图 167　硬腭 Kaposi 肉瘤
Kaposi's sarcoma of the hard palate.

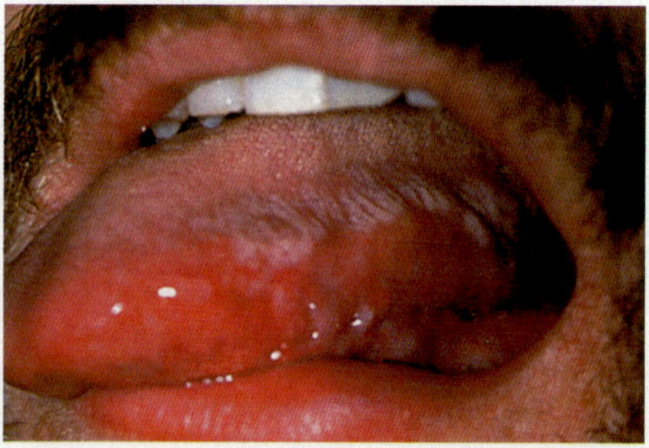

图 168　口腔侧壁毛白斑
Hairy leukoplakia of the lateral border of the tongue.

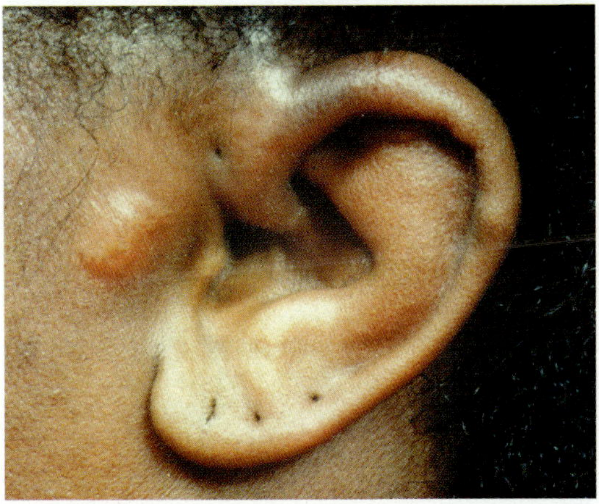

1．这位24岁的女士左耳廓上有4个小孔，最近前面的小孔变得肿胀、疼痛。

a. 这些小孔是什么呢？

b. 她最近的症状如何治疗？

This 24-year-old lady has four small holes in her left pinna. Recently the anterior hole has become swollen and painful.

a. What is the nature of the holes?

b. How should her recent symptoms be managed?

2．这张图片是一患者用棉签“清理”她的耳道。

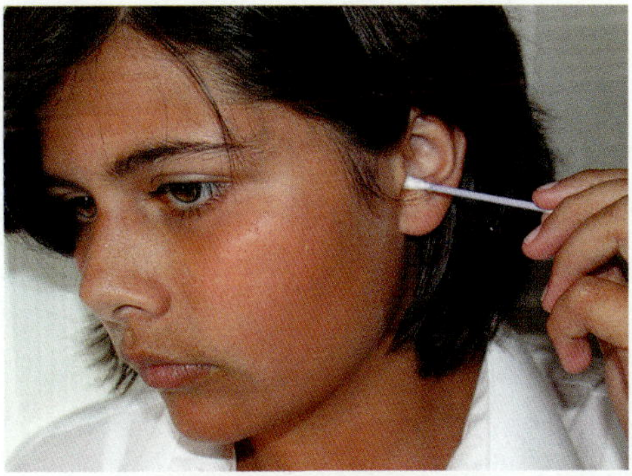

a. 这是清理耵聍的好办法吗？

b. 耵聍是否必须从耳道内清理干净？如果不是，为什么？

c. 用棉签清理耳道的危险是什么？

This photograph shows a patient 'cleaning' her ear with a cotton-tipped applicator.

a. Is this a good way to remove wax from the ear?

b. Does wax have to be removed from the ear? If not, why not?

c. What are the dangers of using cotton-tipped applicators in the ear?

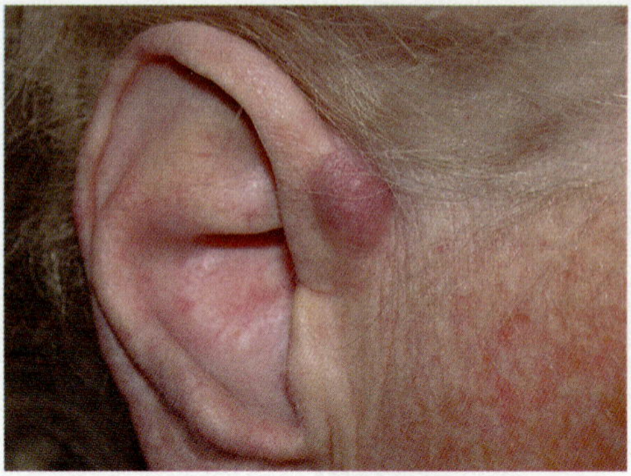

3．图片显示一72岁妇女的右耳廓附近一处病变。该病变充血、肿胀，并且流出脓性分泌物。

a．最可能的诊断是什么?

b．最恰当的治疗是什么?

This photograph shows a lesion near the right pinna of a 72-year-old woman. The lesion has previously become red and swollen, with discharge of purulent material.

a. What is the most likely diagnosis?

b. What is the most appropriate treatment?

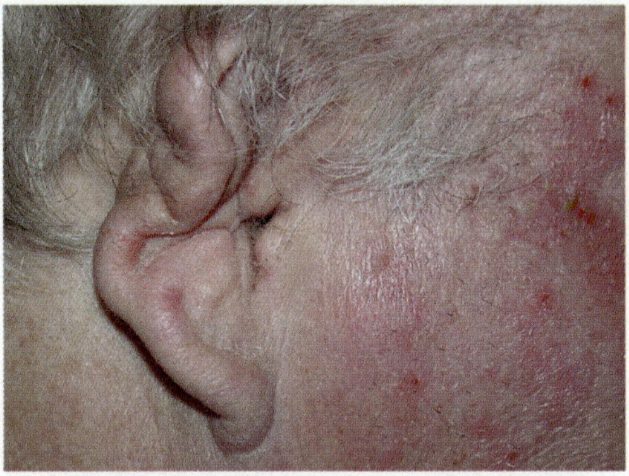

4．这名54岁的男性患者因面部皮疹来医院就诊。他年轻的时候曾打过橄榄球。最近他觉得右耳有刺激感。

a. 描述右耳的外形改变和可能的病理改变。

b. 是什么造成的面部皮疹?

c. 如何治疗?

This 54-year-old man presented to hospital with a facial rash. He used to play rugby football when younger. Recently he has had irritation in his right ear.

a. Describe the appearance of the right ear and the likely pathology.

b. What is the rash caused by?

c. What is the treatment?

5. 这位 11 岁的女孩因单侧传导性聋来耳科就诊。

a. 诊断是什么?

b. 如何治疗?

This 11-year-old girl presented to an ENT clinic with unilateral conductive deafness.

a. What is the diagnosis?

b. What is the treatment?

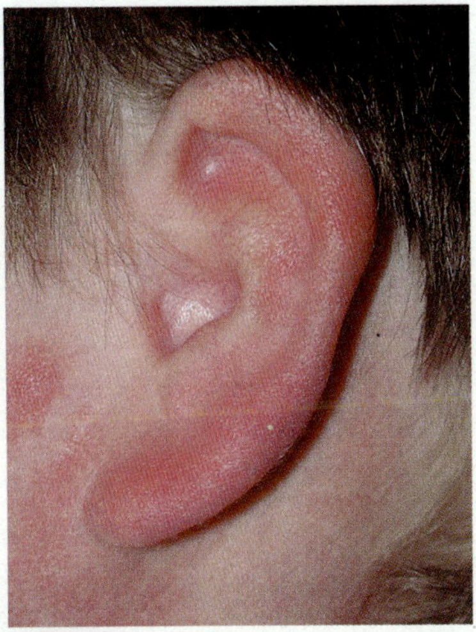

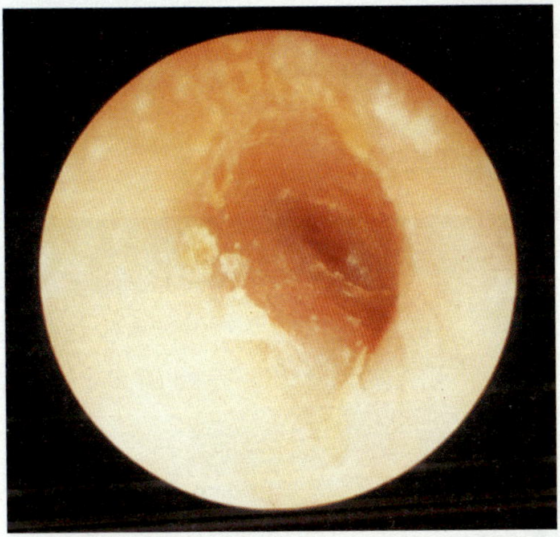

6. 这是一位38岁男性患者耳镜下右耳的局部表现。多年来该患者右耳间断出现耳溢液。近来他觉得听力有所减退。

a. 描述耳镜下所见。

b. 为何会出现这种情况?

c. 如何治疗?

This is the otoscopic appearance of the right ear in a 38-year-old man who has suffered for many years with intermittent aural discharge. Recently he has noticed some difficulty with hearing.

a. Describe the otoscopic appearance.

b. How does this condition arise?

c. What is the treatment?

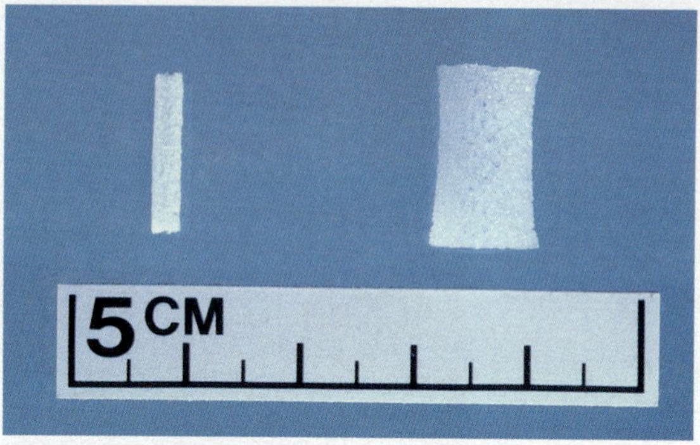

7. 这张图片显示的是治疗耳部疾病所用的填塞物。

a. 何种耳部疾病需用这类填塞物?

b. 用这类填塞物的原则是什么?

This photograph shows a dressing used in the treatment of ear disease.

a. What ear condition is the dressing primarily used for?

b. What is the principle behind the use of this dressing?

8. 这是一位39岁男性患者耳镜下右耳的局部表现。该患者主诉为反复的右耳疼痛和流脓。

a. 诊断是什么?

b. 什么行为导致了这种情况?

c. 如何治疗?

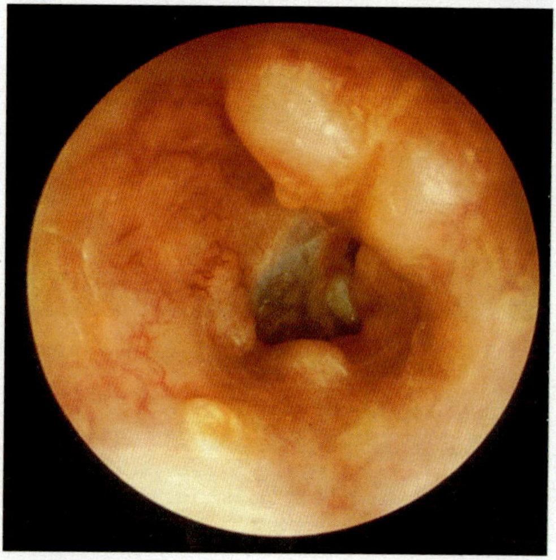

This is the otoscopic appearance of the right ear in a 29-year-old man who suffers with recurrent episodes of pain and discharge from the ear.

a. What is the diagnosis?

b. What activities predispose to the development of this condition?

c. What is the treatment?

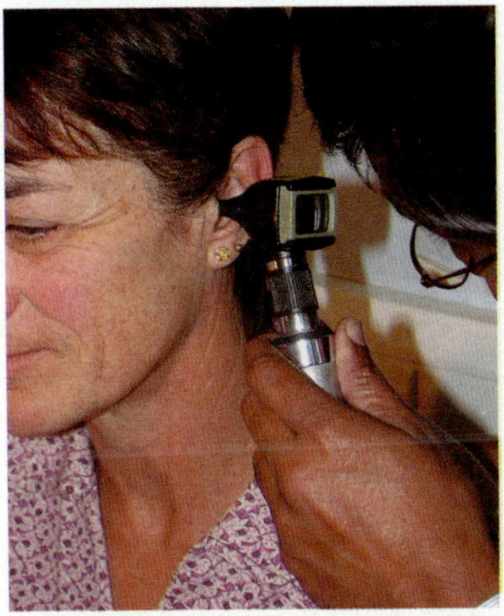
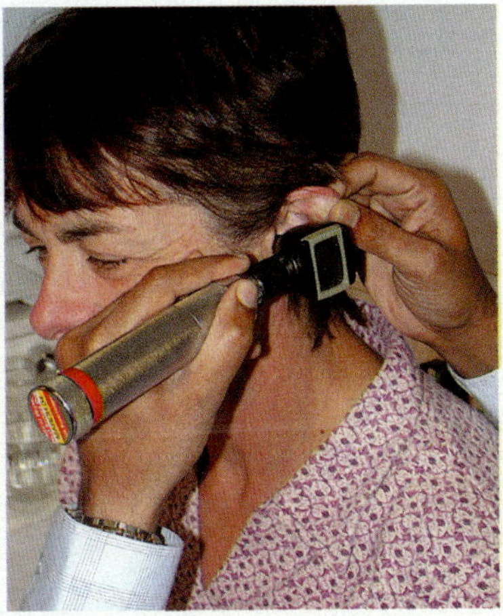

9. 图片显示的是用耳镜检查耳部的两种方法。
哪种方法是正确的？为什么？

These photographs show two ways of examining the ear with an otoscope. Which is the correct method of examination and why?

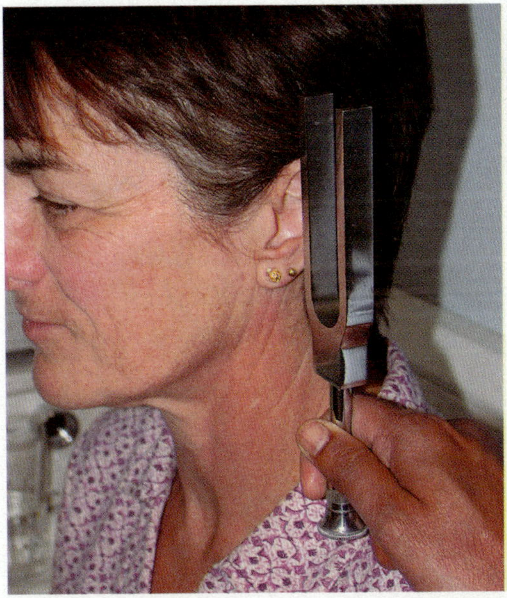
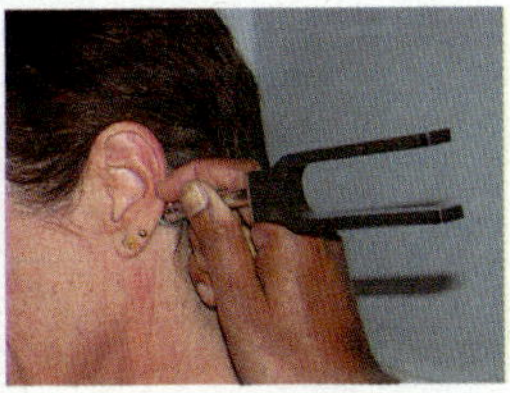

10. 图片显示用音叉试验来评估听力。

a. 这是哪种音叉试验？

b. 用这个试验如何区别不同类型的耳聋？

c. 通常用多少频率的音叉？为什么？

These photographs show a tuning fork being used to assess hearing.

a. What is the name of this particular test?

b. How does this test distinguish between different types of deafness?

c. What is the frequency of the tuning fork usually used and why?

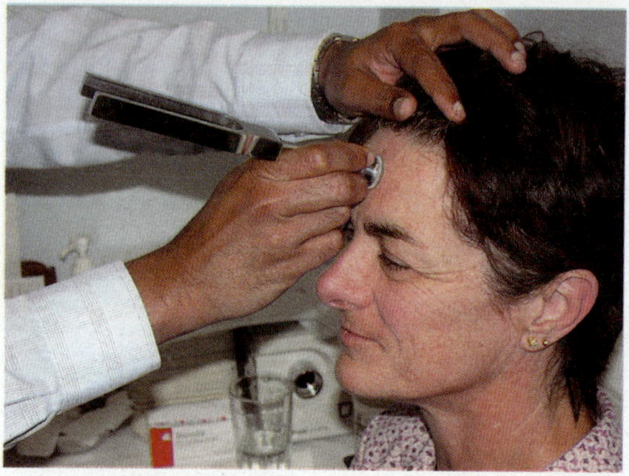

11．图片显示用音叉试验来评估听力。

a. 这是哪种音叉试验？

b. 用这个试验如何区分不同类型的耳聋？

This photograph also shows a tuning fork assessment of hearing.

a. What is the name of this test?

b. How does this distinguish between different types of deafness?

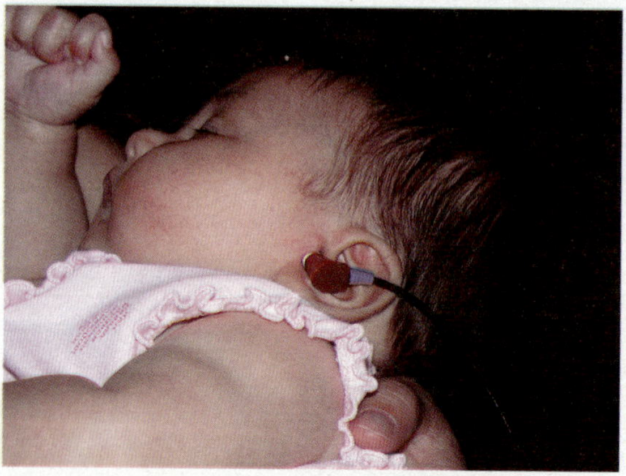

12．图片显示一个新生儿正在接受检查。

a. 这种检查的名称是什么？

b. 这是用于检查什么的？为什么这种检查很重要？

This photograph shows a baby undergoing an investigation in the neonatal period.

a. What is the name of the investigation?

b. What is the investigation designed to establish and why is this important?

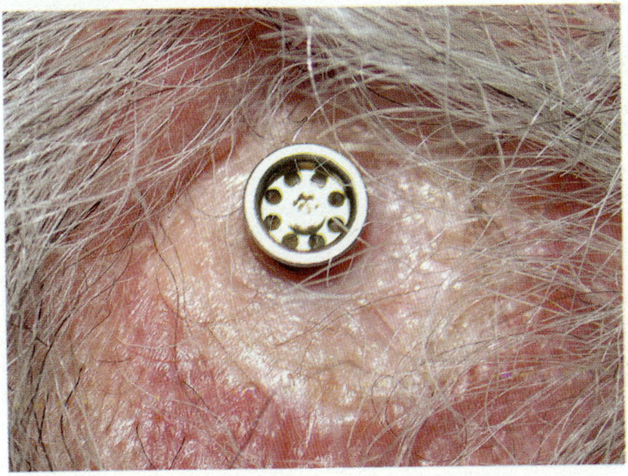

13．这是一名48岁双侧传导性聋的男性患者术后的照片。

a. 他做了什么手术？

b. 为什么要做这种手术？

This photograph shows the healed operation site of a 48-year-old man with bilateral conductive deafness.

a. What operation has been performed?

b. Why has this operation been necessary?

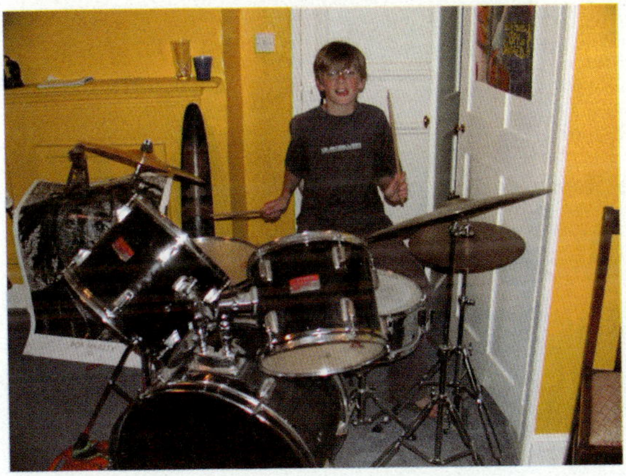

14．这名青少年沉迷于这种娱乐方式。

a. 这种娱乐方式对健康的主要危害是什么？

b. 可能会出现什么症状？

c. 如何治疗？

This teenager is indulging in a hobby.

a. What is the principle health hazard of this pastime?

b. What are the likely symptoms?

c. What is the treatment?

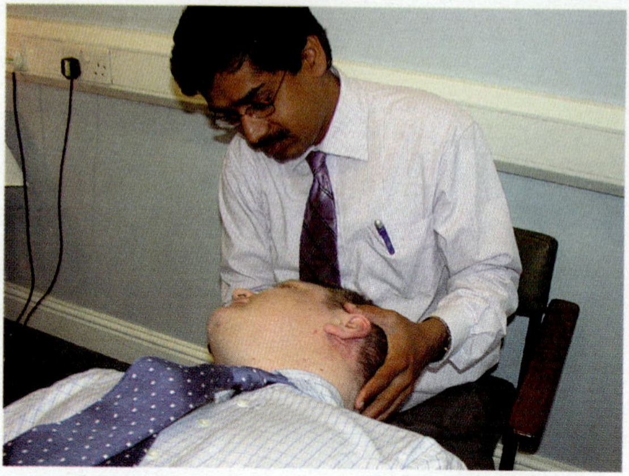

15．这张图片显示的是用于治疗平衡障碍的一种手法。

a. 这是什么手法？用于治疗何种疾病？

b. 这种治疗方法的原理是什么？

This photograph shows a manoeuvre used to treat a disorder of balance.

a. What is the name of this manoeuvre and what condition is being treated?

b. What is the rationale behind this treatment?

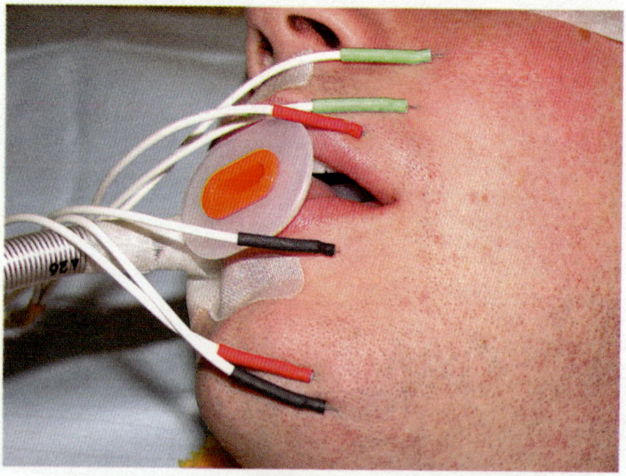

16．这张图片为头颈部手术中行术中监测。

a. 监测的是什么生理功能？

b. 在何种手术当中用到该项监测？

c. 麻醉师应注意什么？

This photograph shows a form of intraoperative monitoring during head and neck surgery.

a. What physiological function is being monitored?

b. During what operations would this equipment be used?

c. What precautions would the anaesthetist need to take?

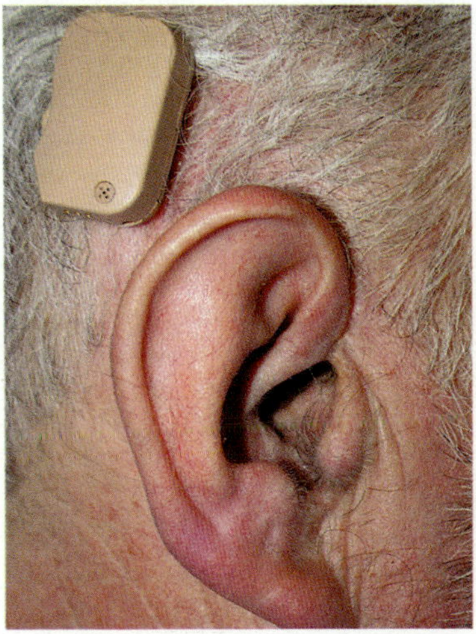

17．这个患者右耳因患胆脂瘤作了手术，术后不能佩戴常规的助听器。

a. 这个患者做了什么手术，为什么术后难以佩戴常规的助听器？

b. 现在这个患者佩戴的是什么助听器？

This patient has had an operation on his right ear for cholesteatoma and finds it difficult to wear a normal conventional hearing aid.

a. What operation was performed for cholesteatoma and why does this make conventional hearing aid use difficult?

b. What type of hearing aid is the patient using?

18．这是一位65岁女性耳聋患者的耳镜表现。其右颈部还有一肿大淋巴结。

a. 诊断是什么？

b. 最可能的潜在病变是什么？

c. 哪个人种最常发生这种情况？

d. 如何治疗？

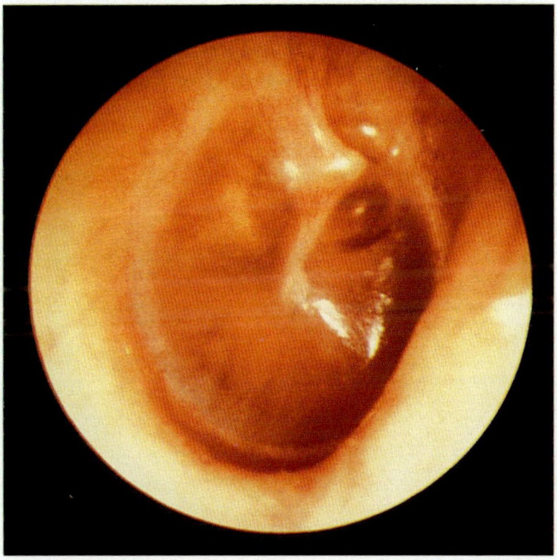

This is the otoscopic appearance of a 65-year-old woman who presents with deafness. She also presents with a mass of lymph nodes on the right side of the neck.

a. What is the diagnosis?

b. What is the most likely underlying pathology?

c. In which racial group is this condition most common?

d. What is the management?

19. 这是一位已多年耳聋的 17 岁男性患者的耳镜检查所见。
a. 描述耳镜检查所见。
b. 过去他有可能接受过怎样的治疗?
c. 现在应当如何治疗?

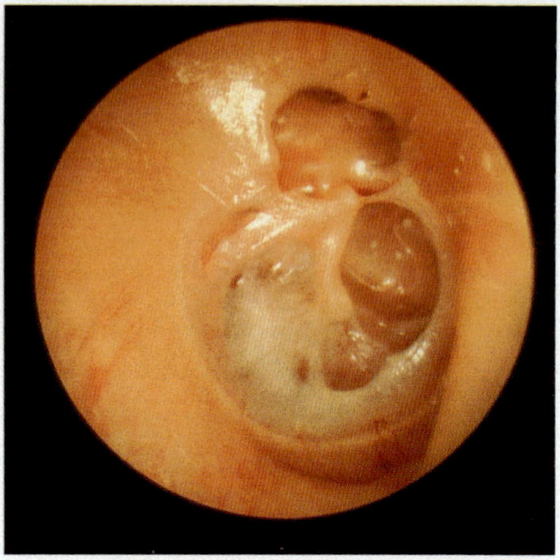

This is the otoscopic appearance of the right ear of a 17-year-old boy who has had hearing problems for many years.

a. Describe the otoscopic features.
b. What type of treatment is he likely to have had in the past?
c. What is the current management?

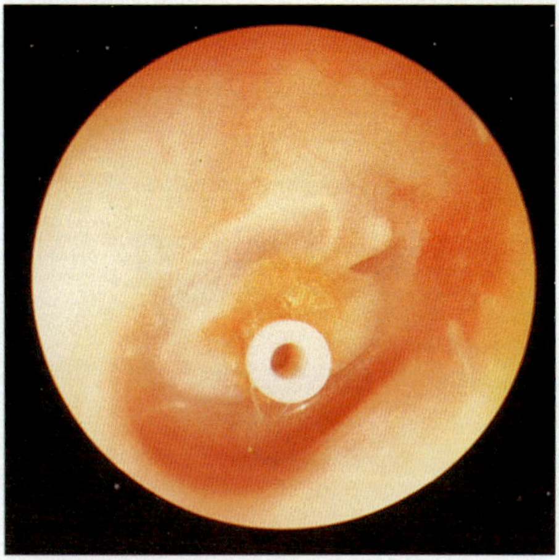

20. 这是一个6岁男孩的耳镜表现，6个月前他曾经做了双耳手术。
a. 他做的是什么手术?
b. 什么情况下应做这种手术?
c. 还有什么其他方法治疗这种疾病?
d. 这个小孩还能游泳吗?

This is the otoscopic appearance of the right ear of a 6-year-old boy who 6 months earlier underwent an operation on both ears.

a. What operation took place?
b. What was the underlying condition for which surgery was necessary?
c. What alternative methods of treatment exist for this condition?
d. Would it be advisable for the child to swim?

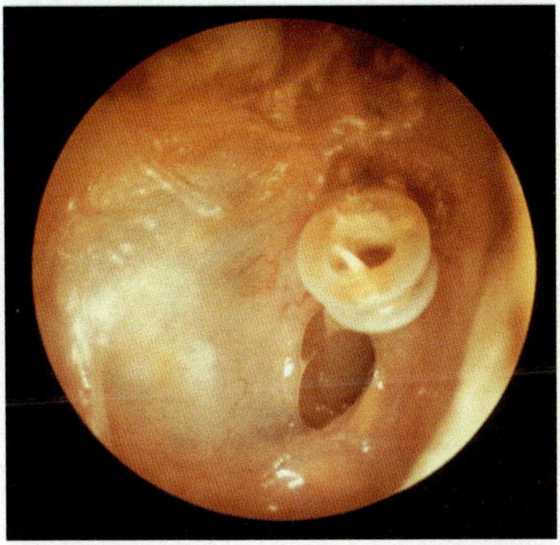

21．这是一个5岁女孩右侧鼓膜的耳镜表现。

a. 描述其耳镜表现。

b. 在此后的三个月有可能出现的情况是什么？

This is the otoscopic appearance of the right tympanic membrane in a 5-year-old girl.

a. Describe the otoscopic features.

b. What is the likely course of events during the following three months?

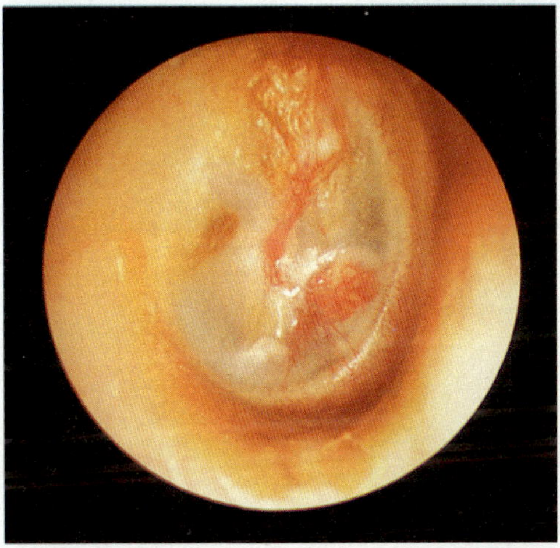

22．这是一位 23 岁男性患者右侧鼓膜的耳镜表现。

a. 诊断是什么？

b. 症状是什么？

c. 如何治疗？

This is the otoscopic appearance of the right tympanic membrane of a 23-year-old man.

a. What is the diagnosis?

b. What are the symptoms?

c. What is the treatment?

23．这是一位23岁男性患者右耳的耳镜表现，他主诉在一次足球赛中右侧头部被撞击后出现耳聋。

a. 诊断是什么？

b. 如何治疗？

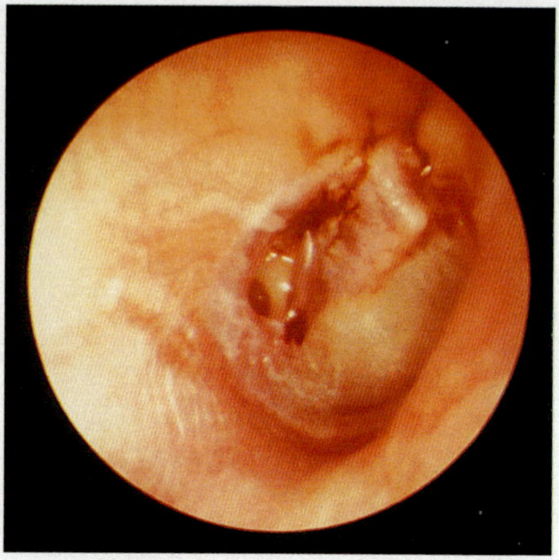

This is the otoscopic appearance of the right ear in a 23-year-old man who complained of deafness following a blow to the side of the head in a soccer match.

a. What is the diagnosis?

b. How is this managed?

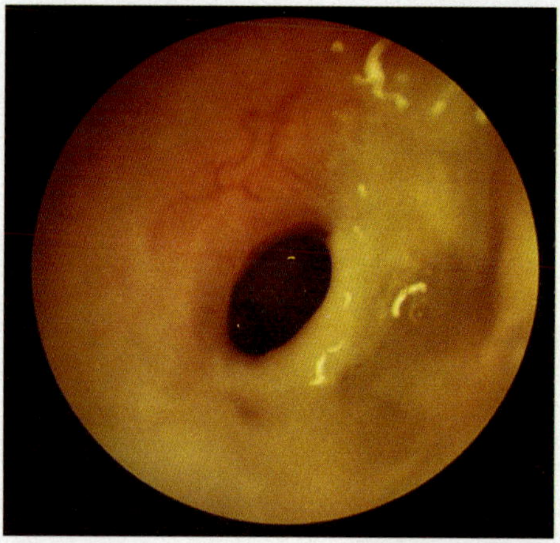

24．这是一位男性患者右侧鼓膜的耳镜表现。在一次配戴水下呼吸器潜水后，他觉得耳内剧痛。几天后开始耳内流脓。

a. 诊断是什么？

b. 最可能的致病微生物是什么？

c. 如何治疗？

This is the otoscopic appearance of the right tympanic membrane of a man who has returned from a scuba diving holiday. During one dive he experienced a sharp pain in his ear. Over the following days he developed a purulent discharge from the ear.

a. What is the diagnosis?

b. What are the microbial organisms most likely to be involved?

c. How is this managed?

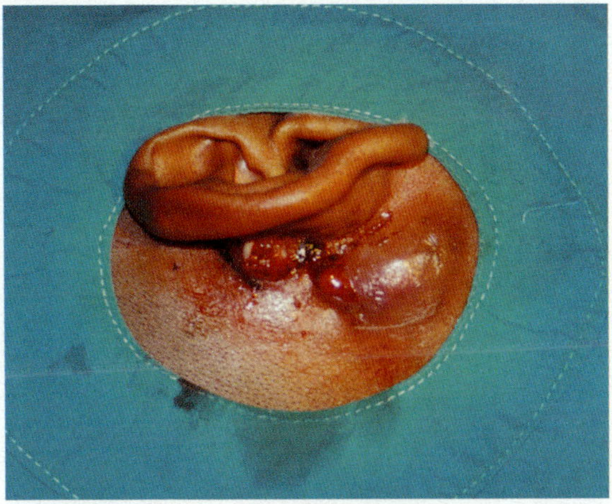

25．这是一位 11 岁的尼泊尔女孩，她已经有两年的耳部症状。

a. 这张图片显示了什么？

b. 最可能的潜在病变是什么？

This is the ear of an 11-year-old Nepali girl presenting with a 2-year history of ear symptoms.

a. What does the photograph show?

b. What is the most likely underlying pathology?

26．这是一位32岁男性患者右耳的耳镜表现，他曾做过中耳手术。

a. 描述其耳镜表现。

b. 他曾做过什么手术？

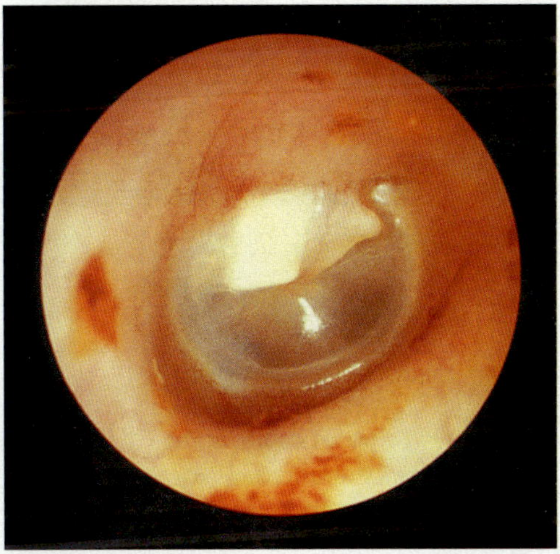

This is the otoscopic appearance of the right ear in a 32-year-old man who has undergone middle ear surgery.

a. Describe the otoscopic appearance

b. What operation has the patient undergone?

27. 这是一位 18 岁女性患者右耳的耳镜表现。
a. 诊断是什么?
b. 在这种情况下，患者常是什么类型的耳聋?
c. 决定耳聋程度的因素是什么?

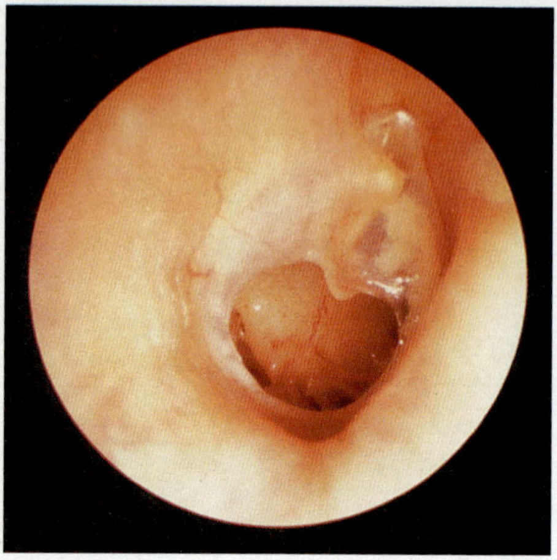

This is the otoscopic appearance of the right ear in an 18-year-old woman.
a. What is the diagnosis?
b. What type of deafness is usually seen in this condition?
c. What factors determine the degree of deafness?

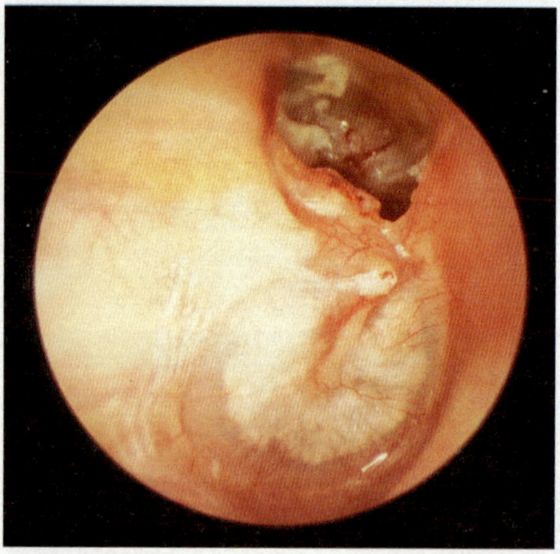

28. 25 岁男性患者，因右耳反复溢液就诊。图为患耳耳镜表现。
a. 诊断是什么?
b. 可能出现哪些并发症?
c. 如何治疗?

This is the otoscopic appearance of the right ear in a 25-year-old man who complained of recurrent discharge from the ear.
a. What is the diagnosis?
b. What are the possible complications of this condition?
c. What is the treatment?

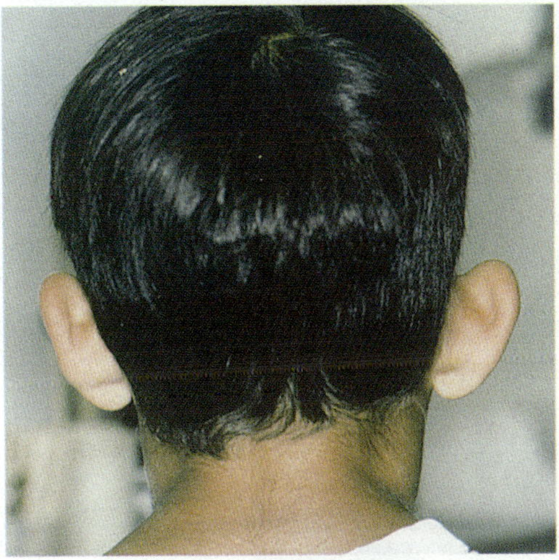

29．这张图片显示的是一位9岁男孩的背面像。注意观察他外耳的表现。

a. 描述其耳部表现。

b. 鉴别诊断是什么？

c. 你将采取何种措施来明确诊断？

This photograph shows the back of a 9-year-old boy's head. Look at the appearance of the external ears.

a. Describe the appearance of the ears.

b. What is the differential diagnosis?

c. What measures would you take to confirm the diagnosis?

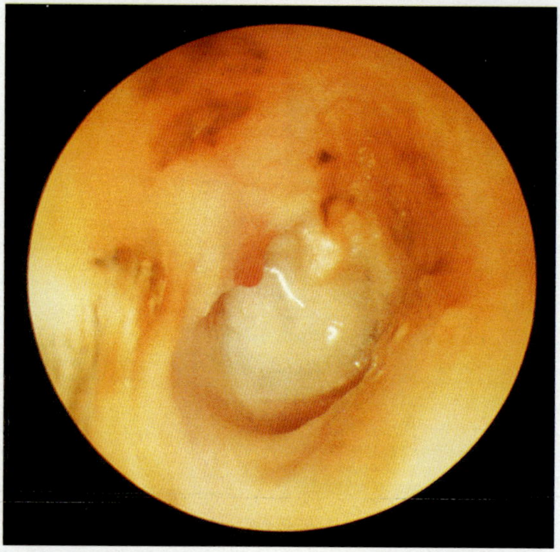

30．这是一位17岁男性患者的耳镜表现，主诉为耳后红肿、疼痛。病史为耳流脓，在他 4 至 11 岁之间曾行 3 次鼓膜置管。

a. 描述其耳镜表现。中耳病变的诊断是什么？

b. 他已经有了什么并发症？

c. 如何治疗并发症及潜在的耳部疾病？

This is the otoscopic appearance of the right ear in a 17-year-old boy who presented with painful red swelling behind the ear. He had a history of discharge from the ear and had undergone grommet insertion on three occasions between the ages of 4 and 11 years.

a. Describe the otoscopic appearance; what is the diagnosis of the middle ear pathology?

b. What complication has arisen?

c. What is the treatment of the complication and the underlying ear disease?

31．这是一位42岁男性患者左耳的耳镜表现，伴有轻度耳聋和耳流脓。

a. 诊断是什么？

b. 通过图片你可以看到哪部分的中耳听骨链？

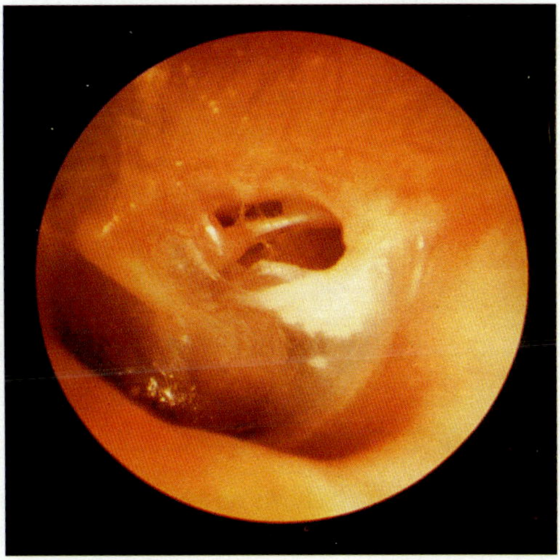

This is the otoscopic appearance of the left ear in a 42-year-old man with mild deafness and occasional discharge from the ear.

a. What is the diagnosis?

b. What parts of the middle ear ossicular chain are visible?

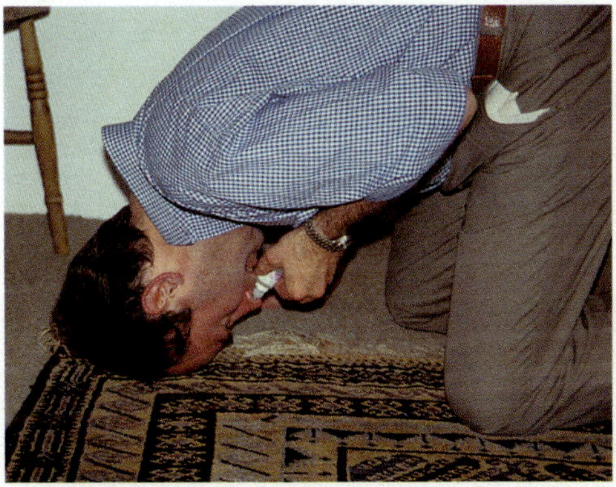

32．中年男性患者，自行鼻内用药。

a. 这可能是用了哪类药物？

b. 患者为什么要采取这种体位？

c. 在什么情况下要采取这种体位？

d. 这类治疗方式的危害是什么？

This middle-aged man is self-administering nasal medication.

a. What is the likely nature of the medication?

b. Why is the patient adopting this position?

c. What conditions are treated in this way?

d. What are the dangers of this medication?

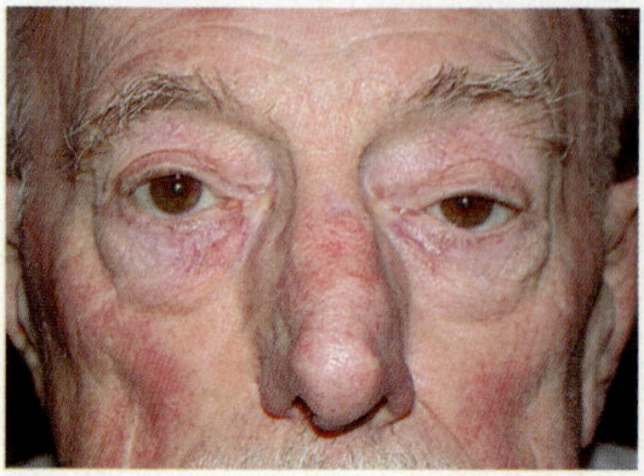
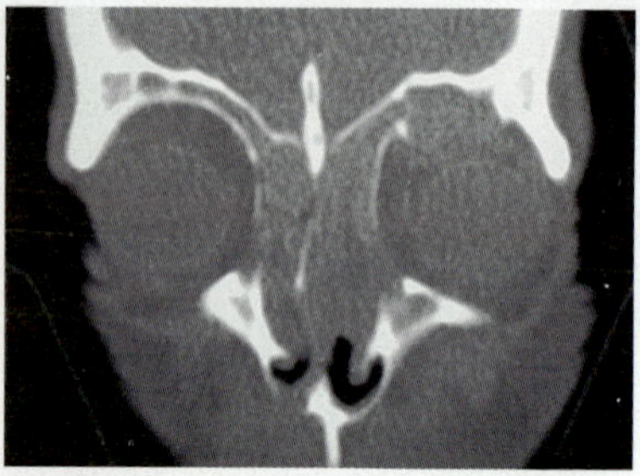

33. 82 岁男性患者的照片和相应的鼻窦 CT。主诉：近来有复视。

a. 描述其临床表现。

b. 描述鼻窦 CT 情况，解释鼻窦病变引起复视的原因。

This photograph shows an 82-year-old man with a recent onset of double vision (diplopia). His corresponding sinus CT scan is also shown.

a. Describe the clinical appearance.

b. What dose the sinus CT show and how has the sinus pathology caused the diplopia?

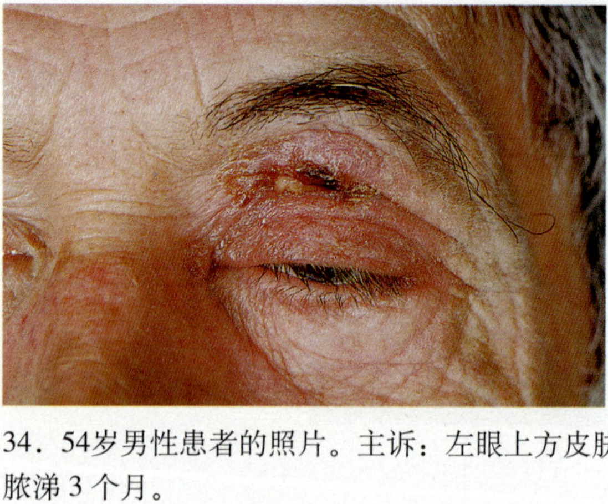

34. 54岁男性患者的照片。主诉：左眼上方皮肤破溃流脓伴鼻堵、脓涕 3 个月。

a. 皮肤破溃流脓与鼻部症状的关系是什么？

b. 该病如何处理？

This photograph shows a 54-year-old man with a discharging lesion above the left eye. He also complains of nasal stuffiness and purulent nasal discharge, present for 3 months.

a. How might the discharging lesion be related to the nasal symptoms?

b. How should this case be managed?

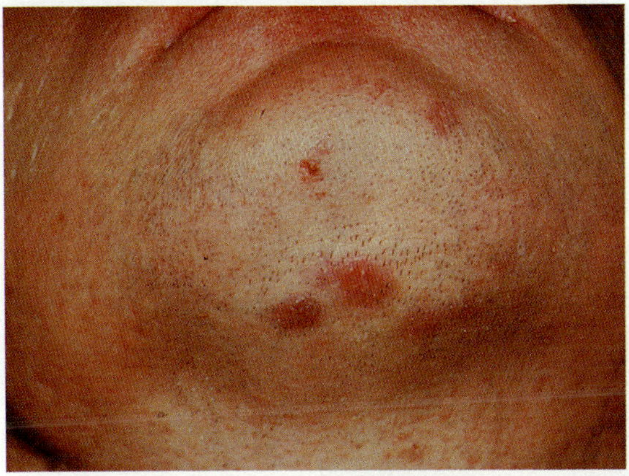

35．44岁男性患者面部皮肤病变的照片。该患者人类免疫缺陷病毒（HIV）抗体阳性。

a. 皮肤病变的诊断是什么？

b. 怎样治疗面部的皮肤病变？

This photograph shows lesions on the facial skin in a 44-year-old man who has positive antibodies for human immunodeficiency virus (HIV).

a. What is the diagnosis of the facial lesions?

b. What is the treatment of the facial lesions?

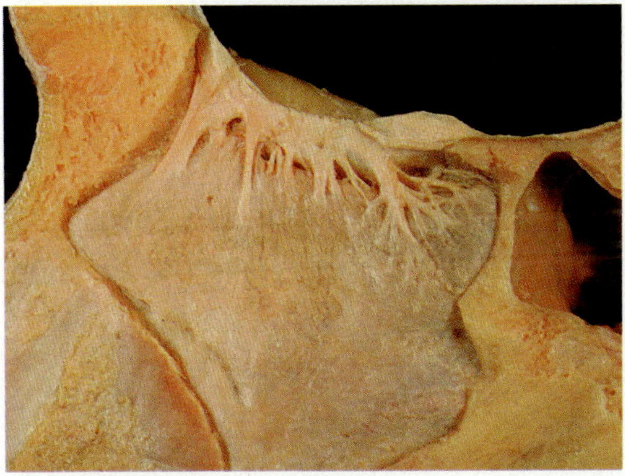

36．尸解矢状切面显示鼻中隔。

a. 哪些解剖结构组成鼻中隔？

b. 鼻中隔上方的丝状结构是什么？它们的功能是什么？

This cadaver section shows the nasal septum.

a. What anatomical structures form the nasal septum?

b. What are the filamentous structures at the top of the septum and what is their function?

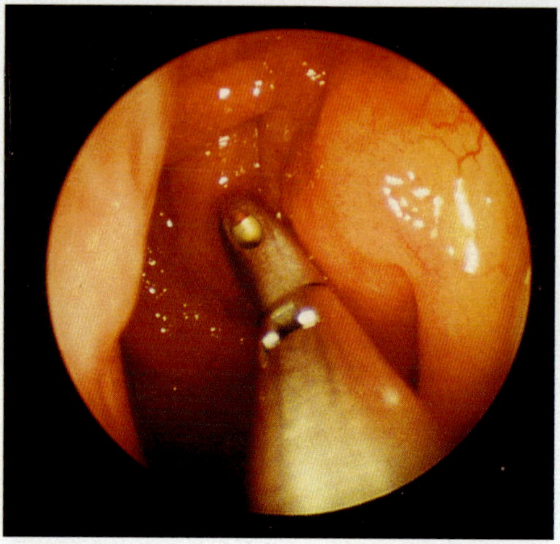

37．54 岁男性患者，主诉：颈部肿块和单侧耳聋。图为鼻内镜下鼻咽部的活检。

a. 鼻咽部的病理可能是什么？哪类人群易患这种疾病？

b. 为什么会出现颈部肿块和单侧耳聋？

This is an endoscopic view of a biopsy being taken from the nasopharynx in a 54-year-old male presenting with a lump in the neck and unilateral deafness.

a. What pathology is suspected in the nasopharynx and what population group is particularly likely to suffer from this condition?

b. Explain the lump in the neck and unilateral deafness.

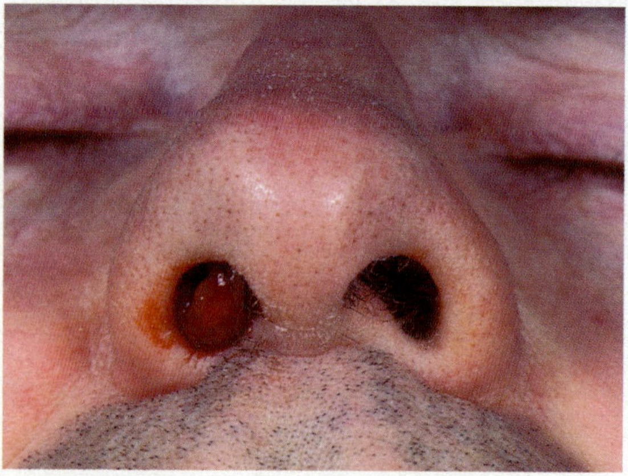

38．67 岁男性患者的鼻部照片。

a. 描述它的表现。

b. 鉴别诊断是什么？

c. 哪些症状应疑为严重病变？

This photograph shows the nose of a 67-year-old man.

a. Describe the appearance.

b. What is the differential diagnosis?

c. What symptoms would suggest serious pathology?

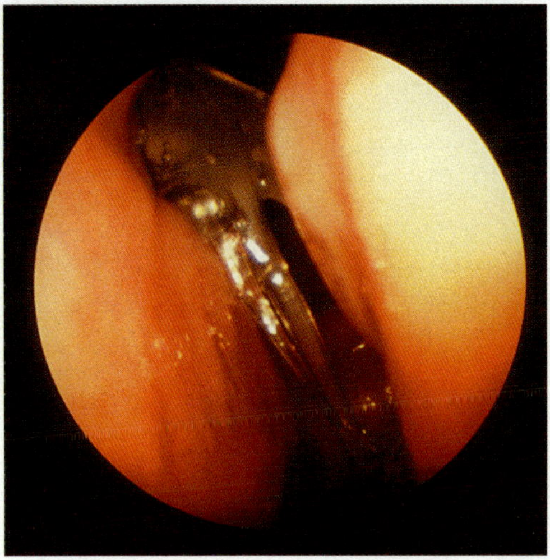

39．患者主诉“卡他”。图为鼻内镜下的鼻腔表现。

a. 描述内镜所见和“卡他”的性质。

b. 如何处理“卡他”症状？

This photograph shows the endoscopic appearance of the nasal cavity in a patient complaining of 'catarrh'.

a. Describe the endoscopic appearance, and the nature of 'catarrh'.

b. What can be done about this symptom?

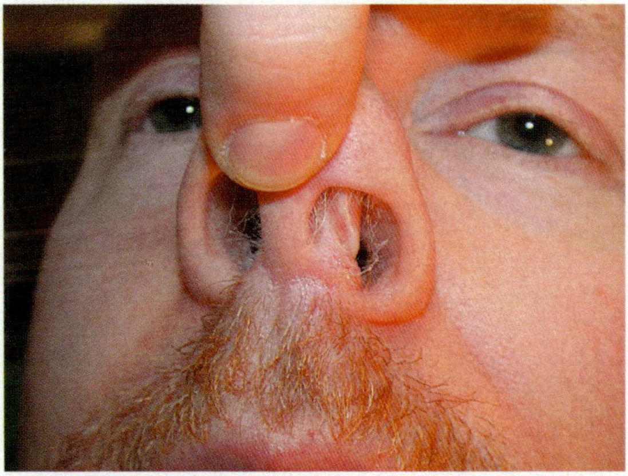

40．鼻堵患者的鼻部照片。

a. 鼻堵的原因是什么？

b. 怎样治疗？

This photograph shows the nose of a patient with nasal blockage.

a. What is the cause of the nasal blockage?

b. What treatment would be possible?

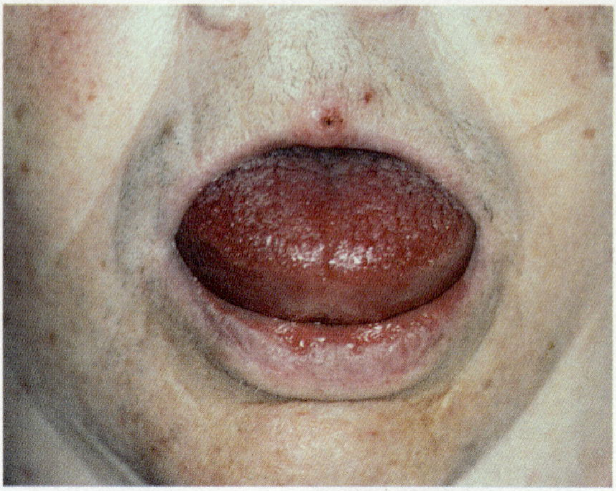

41．63 岁女性患者，因外伤致舌急性肿胀。

a. 鉴别诊断是什么?

b. 如何保持呼吸道通畅?

c. 急诊处理时应用何药?

This photograph shows the tongue of a 63-year-old lady who presented to an accident and emergency department with an acute onset of tongue swelling.

a. What is the differential diagnosis?

b. What airway support would be appropriate?

c. What drugs might be used in the acute treatment?

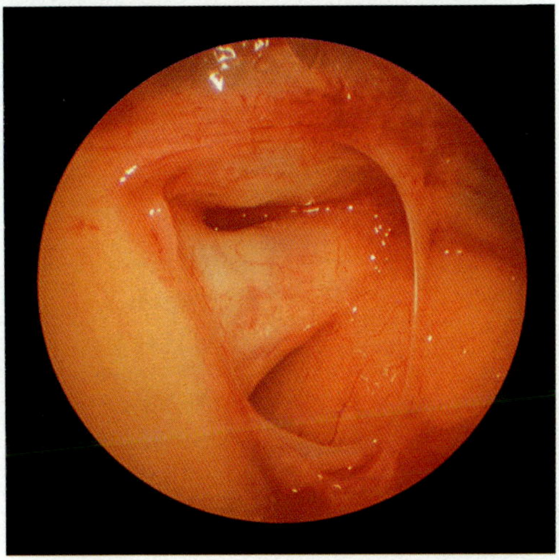

42．鼻窦内镜手术显示蝶窦内的结构，如果损伤这些结构可引起严重并发症。

a. 所显示的结构是什么？

b. 在鼻窦内镜手术中，还有哪些结构损伤后会引起严重并发症？

This is the endoscopic view of a structure seen in the sphenoid sinus during endoscopic sinus surgery, damage to which would result in a major complication.

a. What is the structure shown?

b. What other structures can be damaged by ENT surgeons in the sinuses, leading to major complications?

43．23岁男性患者，右眼击伤后出现复视。图为CT扫描情况。

a. 描述CT表现，这种特殊外伤通常称什么？

b. 怎样治疗复视？

This is the CT scan of a 23-year-old man who was punched in the right eye. Following the injury he complained of double vision.

a. What does the CT scan show and by what name is this particular injury usually known by?

b. What is the treatment for the man's double vision?

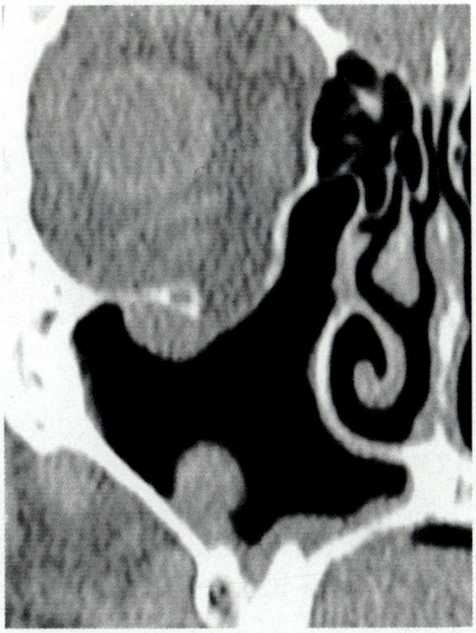

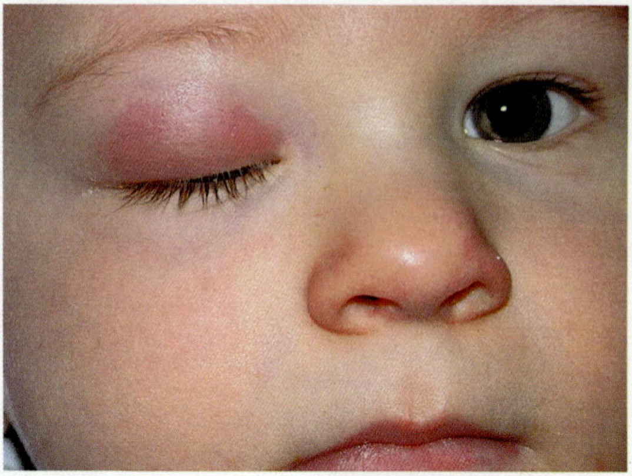

44．2岁患儿，因上呼吸道感染后出现右眼周肿胀 3 天。

a. 诊断是什么？

b. 病因是什么？

c. 怎样治疗？ 如果治疗不及时，后果是什么？

This is a 2-year-old child with a 3-day history of swelling around the right eye following an upper respiratory tract infection.

a. What is the diagnosis?

b. What is the cause of this condition?

c. What is the treatment, and what would the natural history of the condition be if untreated?

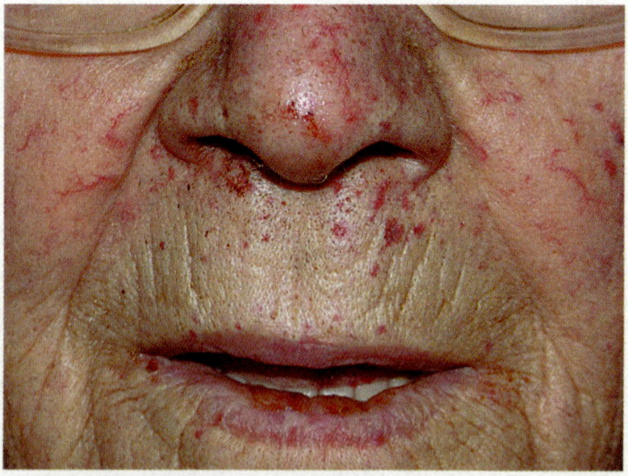

45．80岁老年男性患者的面部照片，主因反复鼻出血而多次住院治疗。他的儿女及兄弟都有类似病史。

a. 这是什么病？

b. 它的遗传方式是什么？

c. 应该怎样治疗这种情况下的鼻出血？

This is a photograph of an 80-year-old man suffering with recurrent epistaxis requiring repeated admission to hospital. His son, daughter and brother also have the condition.

a. What is the condition?

b. What is the mode of inheritance?

c. What is the treatment of the epistaxis associated with this condition?

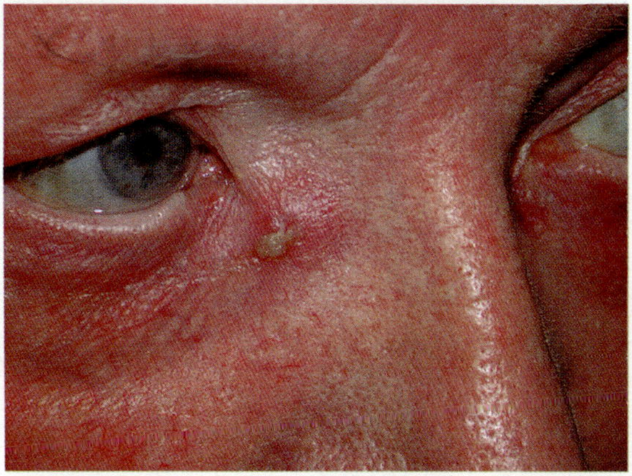

46．74 岁女性患者，近右眼处有一窦道流脓，右眼溢泪。

a. 最可能的诊断是什么？

b. 如何治疗？

This 74-year-old woman has a discharging sinus close to her right eye. She also complains of a watery right eye.

a. What is the most likely diagnosis?

b. What is the appropriate treatment?

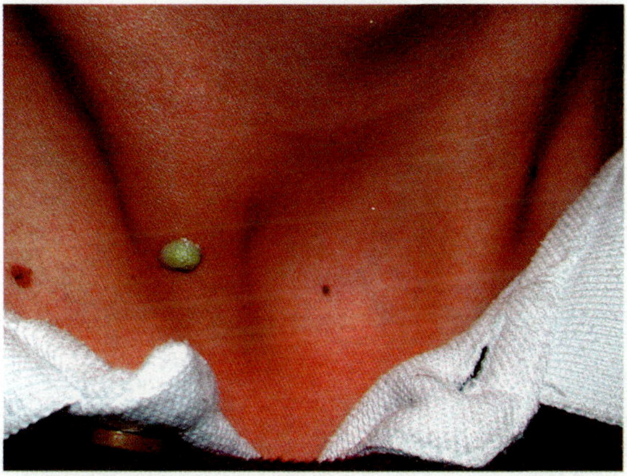

47．14 岁男孩，自幼颈部有一窦道反复流脓。

a. 诊断是什么？

b. 如何处理？

This 14-year-old boy presented with a lesion in his neck that had been discharging purulent material since early childhood.

a. What is the diagnosis?

b. What is the treatment?

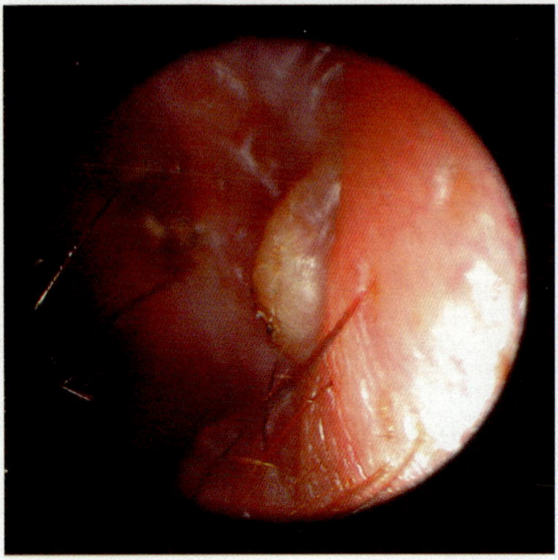

48. 图为内镜显示的鼻前庭病变，该男性患者24岁，手指上有类似病变。

a. 病变是什么?

b. 病因是什么?

c. 是癌前病变吗?

d. 如何治疗?

This is an endoscopic photograph showing a lesion in the nasal vestibule of a 24-year-old man. The man has similar lesions on his fingers.

a. What is the lesion?

b. What is the aetiological agent?

c. Is the lesion pre-malignant?

d. What is the treatment?

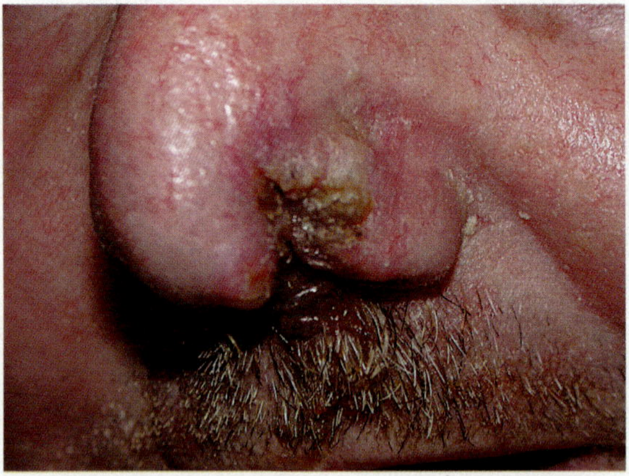

49. 70 岁男性患者的鼻部照片，外鼻有病变。

a. 鉴别诊断是什么?

b. 怎样治疗?

This is a photograph of a 70-year-old man with a lesion of the external nose.

a. What is the differential diagnosis?

b. What is the treatment?

50．患者男，19岁，在英国每年夏季鼻部症状发作。图为鼻内镜下鼻腔情况。

a. 照片显示什么问题？

b. 可能的诊断及诱发因素是什么？

c. 如何治疗？

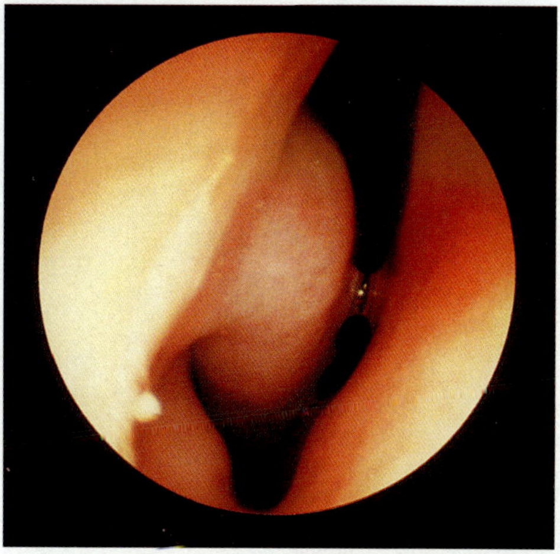

This is an endoscopic photograph of the nasal cavity of a 19-year-old man who suffers with nasal symptoms during the summer months in the UK.

a. What does the photograph show?

b. What is the likely diagnosis and what are the likely causative factors?

c. What is the treatment?

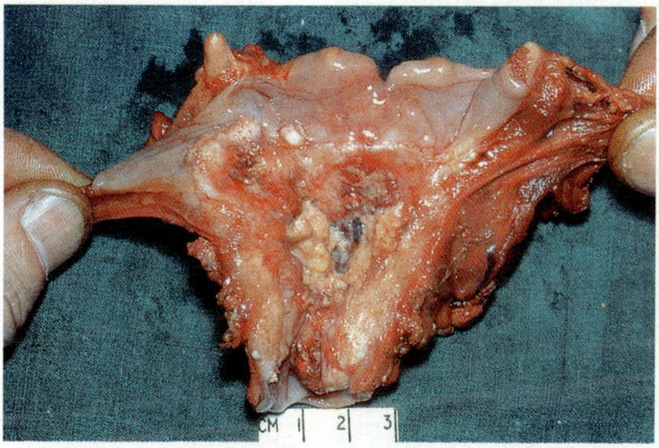

51．图为手术切除标本。

a. 这是什么器官？什么疾病？

b. 该病的病因是什么？

c. 该病变通常如何扩展？

d. 最适宜的治疗方案是什么？

This photograph is of a surgical resection specimen.

a. What is the structure and disease demonstrated?

b. What is the aetiology of this disease?

c. How does it usually spread?

d. What treatment modalities are appropriate for it?

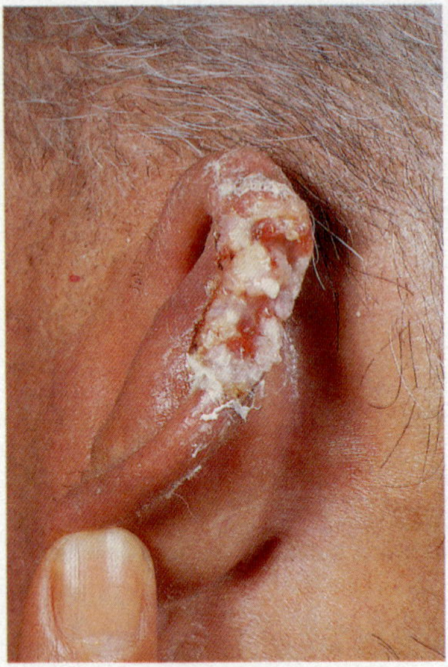

52．图为一位75岁男性患者左耳轮部溃疡性病变。

a. 最可能的病理诊断是什么？

b. 若不治疗，疾病将如何发展？

c. 适宜的治疗方案是什么？

d. 可能的病因是什么？

This is the ulcerated pinna of a 75-year-old man.

a. What is the likely pathological diagnosis?

b. Left untreated, how is the disease likely to progress?

c. What modes of treatment are appropriate?

d. What is the probable aetiology?

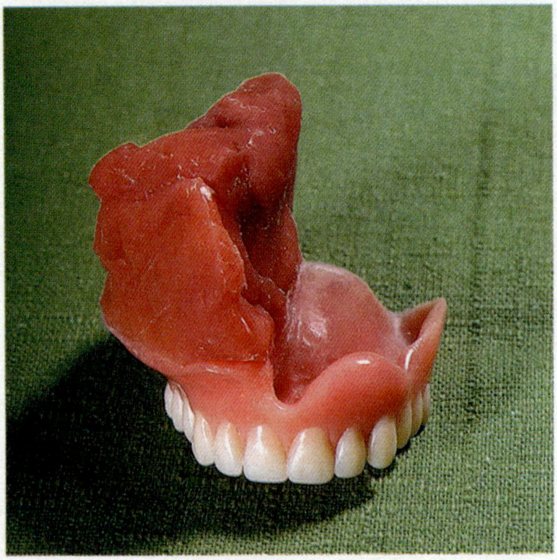

53．图为一上列牙托。

a. 患者经受了什么手术？

b. 什么是溢泪？

c. 此类疾病是早期病例多见还是晚期病例多见？

This prosthesis consists of a dental plate and obturator.

a. What procedure has the patient undergone?

b. What is epiphora?

c. Do such lesions usually present early or late?

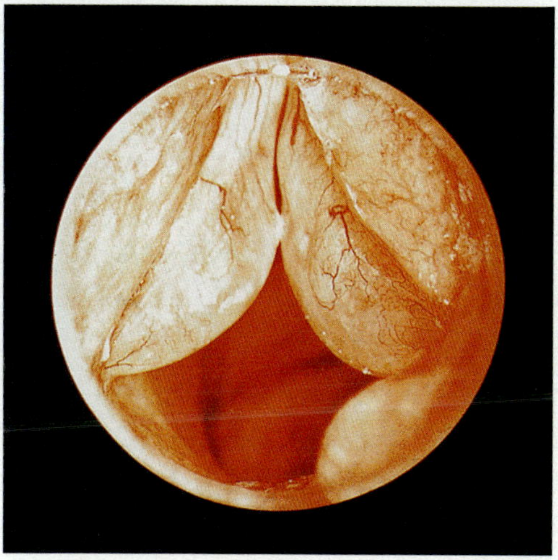

54．图为一 44 岁女性喉部的内镜照片。

a. 这是一个典型的什么病变？

b. 可能的病因是什么？

c. 你认为该如何治疗？

This is the endoscopic appearance of the larynx of a 44-year-old woman.

a. What is this a typical example of?

b. What are the possible aetiologies?

c. How would you treat the condition?

55．一位65岁长期吸烟斗的患者的舌外观。

a. 诊断及病因是什么？

b. 这种病情严重吗？

c. 如何治疗？

d. 舌癌的常见表现是什么？

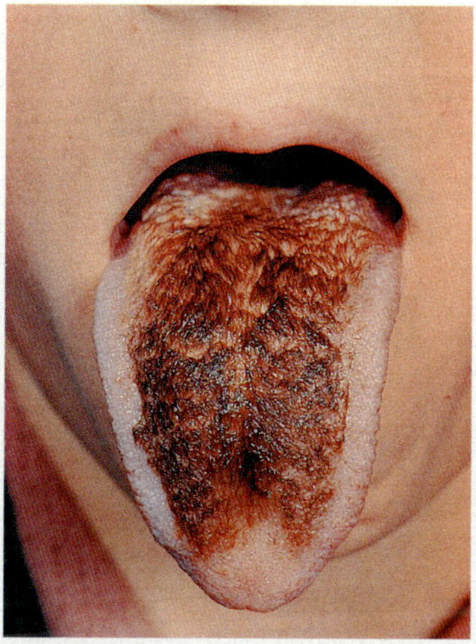

A 65-year-old pipe-smoker is worried about the appearance of his tongue.

a. What is the diagnosis and its cause?

b. Is the condition serious?

c. How is it treated?

d. How do tongue cancers usually present?

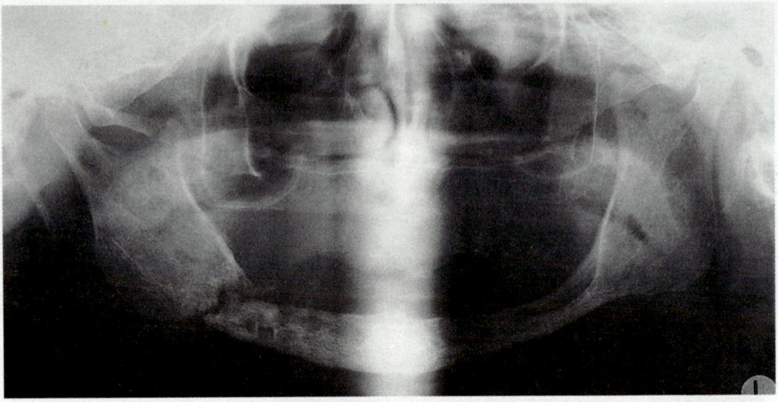

56．一位男性患者因下颌骨牙槽附近溃疡就诊。图为该患者的X线片。

a. 这是哪种 X 线片？

b. 此时这种平片为何特别有用？

c. 本例中，它提示什么疾病？

d. 若病理提示恶性肿瘤，那么放疗适合吗？

This is an X-ray of the mandible of a man who presents with an ulcer adjacent to the right lower alveolus.

a. What type of X-ray is this?

b. Why is it particularly useful?

c. What does it demonstrate in this instance?

d. If a biopsy demonstrates a malignancy would radiotherapy be an appropriate treatment?

57．37岁女性，颈中部肿胀一年。

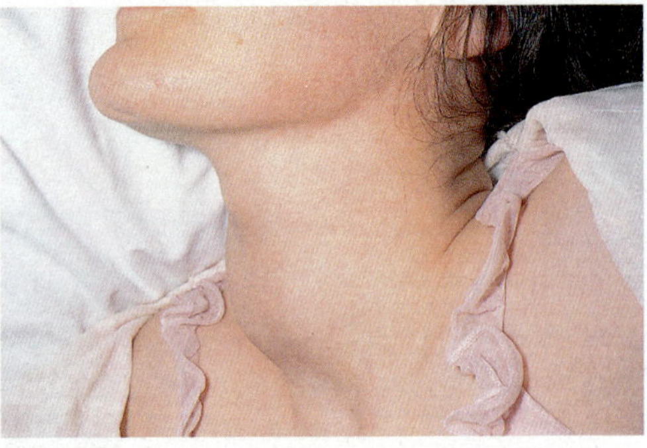

a. 可能的疾病是什么？

b. 该病良性与恶性哪个可能性大？

c. 你认为还应如何进一步检查？

d. 你应该要着重询问哪些症状？

A 37-year-old lady presents with a year's history of a midline neck swelling.

a. What is the probable cause?

b. Is the underlying process likely to be benign or malignant?

c. How would you investigate the problem?

d. What particular symptoms would you ask about?

58．该患者患有右侧颊部皮肤的血管畸形。

a. 这种表现常见于什么综合征？

b. 该综合征还有什么表现？

c. 患者可有哪些症状？

This patient has a vascular malformation of the skin of the right cheek.

a. What syndrome does this almost certainly form part of?

b. What are its other facets?

c. What are the resulting symptoms?

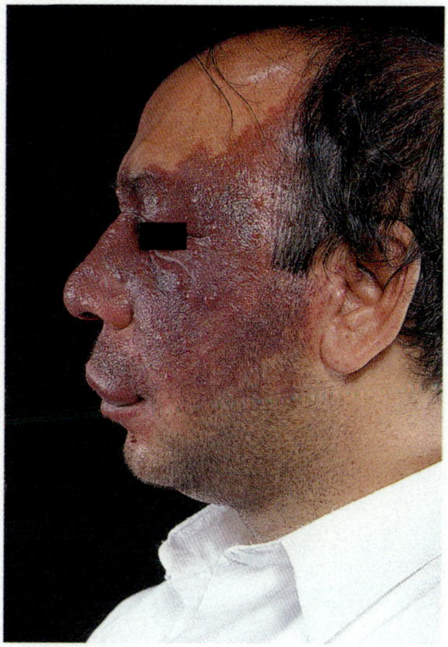

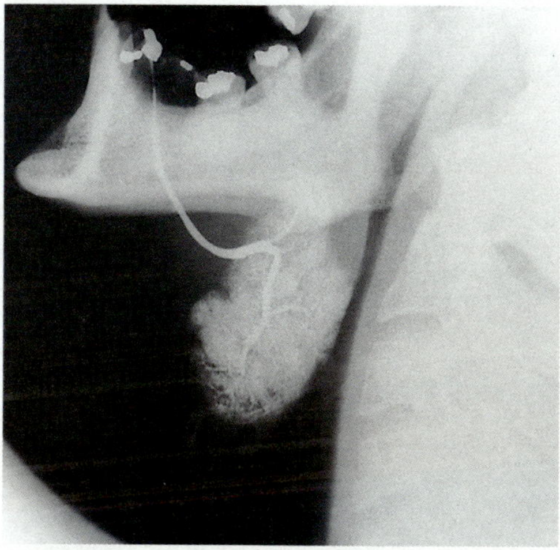

59．这是一位 50 岁男性的口腔及上颈部 X 片。

a. 还应作什么检查？

b. 该病最可能出现什么症状？

c. 该片中有何异常表现？

d. 该结构附近有什么神经？

This is the X-ray of the oral cavity and upper neck of a 50-year-old man.

a. What investigation is being undertaken?

b. What are the likely symptoms necessitating it?

c. What specific abnormalities can the test demonstrate?

d. What nerves lie in close proximity to the structure?

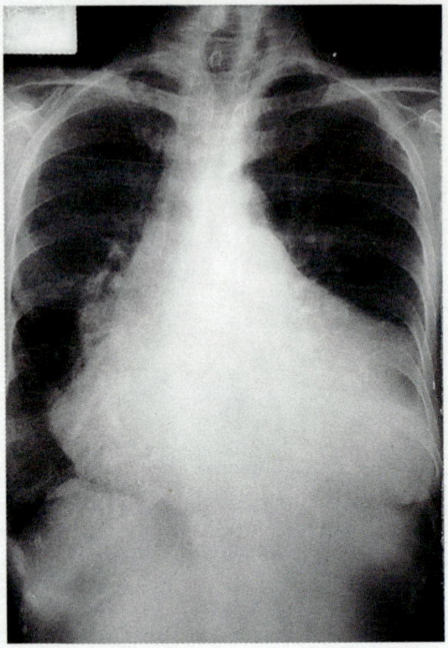

60．男性患者，76 岁，有声嘶。图为该患者胸片。

a. 该疾病的发病过程是什么？

b. 患者为什么会有声嘶？

c. 还可有什么症状？

d. 如何治疗？

This is the chest X-ray of a 76-year-old man with a hoarse voice.

a. What is the disease process?

b. Why is he hoarse?

c. What other symptoms should be sought?

d. What is the treatment of these symptoms?

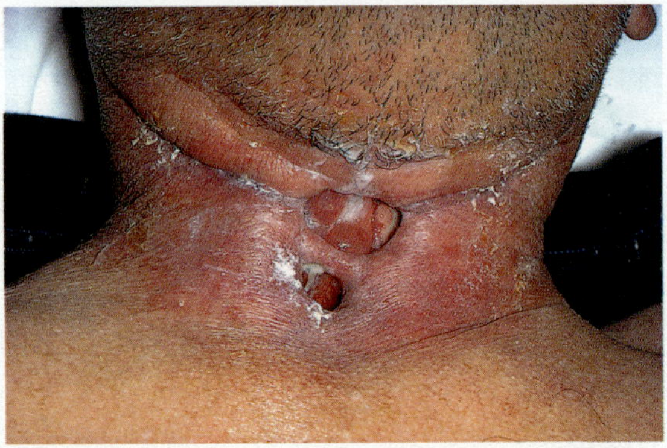

61．喉癌喉全切除术后 3 周，颈部可见两个“洞”。

a. 位于下方的“洞”是什么？

b. 上方的“洞”可能与什么部位相通？

c. 此种头颈部大手术后伤口破损特别常见于哪类患者？

This man underwent a laryngectomy for advanced cancer three weeks prior to this photograph. There are two distinct 'holes' in the neck skin.

a. What is the lower one?

b. With what structure does the upper one probably communicate?

c. Which particular patients are at risk of such wound breakdown following major head and neck surgery?

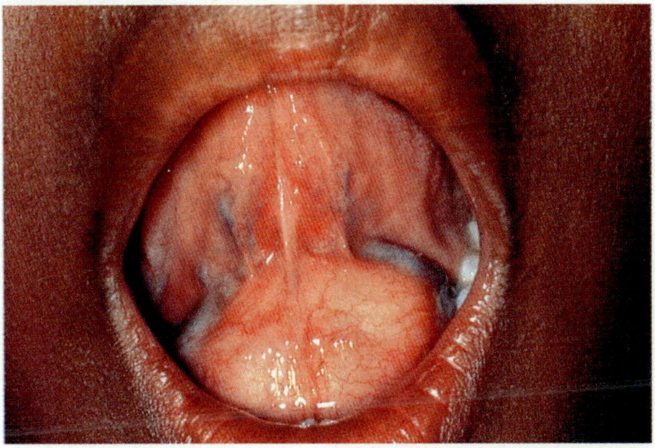

62．一位口底肿胀的女性患者。

a. 如何判断肿胀为实性还是囊性？

b. 此时最应行何种检查？

c. 可能出现什么并发症？

This lady has a swelling of the floor of her mouth.

a. Clinically how would you decide whether it was solid or cystic?

b. What investigation would be most helpful?

c. Are there any specific complications which can result from swellings at this site?

63．长期气管插管可造成声带损伤，以至于拔管后声嘶、呼吸困难。

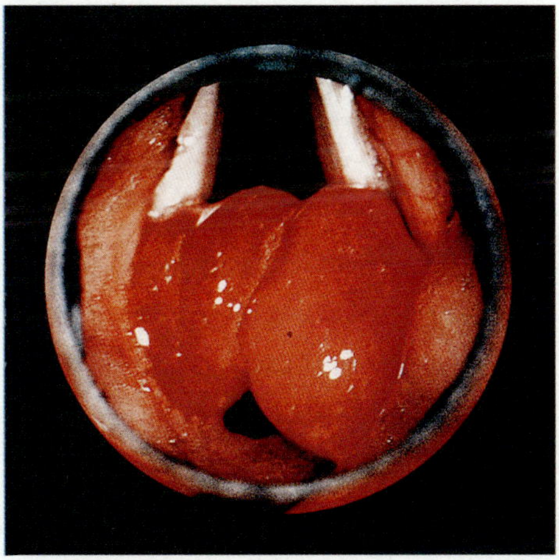

a. 该并发症的病理基础是什么？

b. 如何避免这种情况发生？

c. 最佳治疗手段是什么？

Prolonged endotracheal intubation can result in vocal cord damage with hoarseness and airway compromise following extubation.

a. What is the pathological process involved in this instance?

b. How can this situation be avoided?

c. How is it best treated?

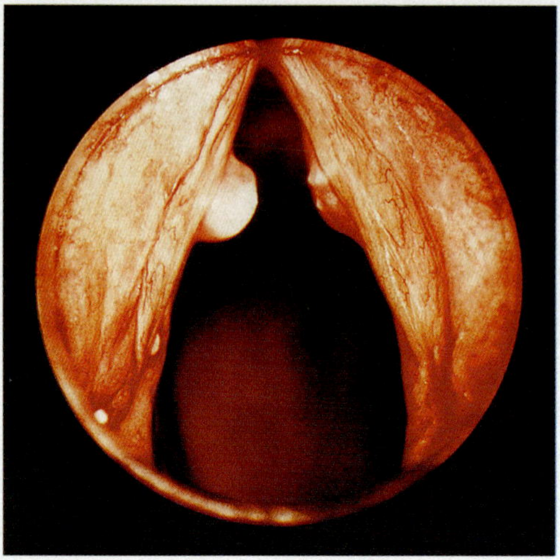

64．45 岁教师，不吸烟。图为其喉部照片。

a. 诊断是什么？

b. 治疗方案是什么？

c. 如何预防该病？

This is the larynx of a 45-year-old non-smoking schoolteacher.

a. What is the diagnosis?

b. How is it treated?

c. How can it be avoided?

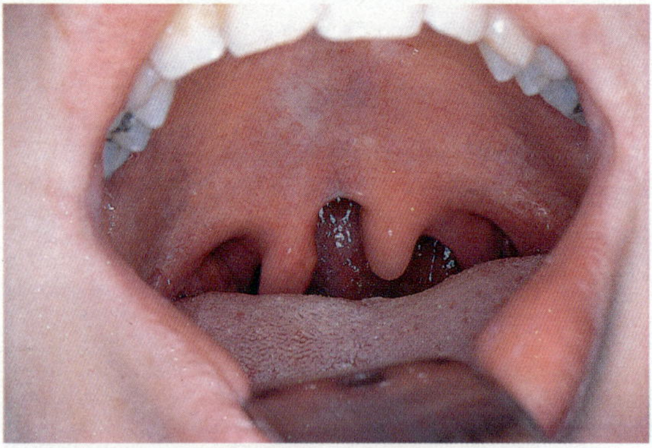

65．男童，以鼻堵就诊。图为其口咽部外观。

a. 这张图片有何异常？

b. 该病常见于什么情况？

c. 应避免对该患者行什么手术？

This is the appearance of the oropharynx of a boy with a history of nasal obstruction.

a. What does this slide demonstrate?

b. What could this be associated with?

c. Are there any surgical procedures that should be avoided?

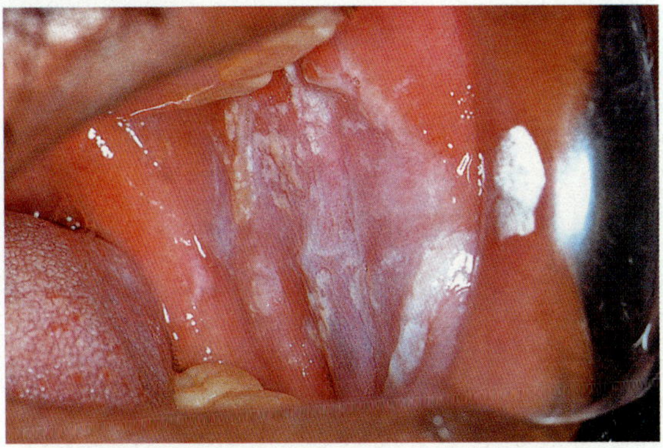

66. 图为一位 55 岁女性患者的颊黏膜外观。

a. 这是什么疾病?

b. 如何确诊?

c. 如何治疗?

This is the appearance of the buccal mucosa of a 55-year-old female.

a. What is the clinical condition?

b. How would you confirm the diagnosis?

c. What is the treatment?

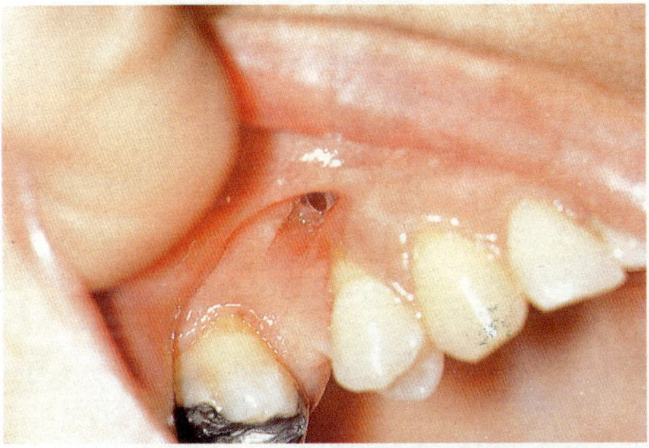

67. 患者于牙科手术后诉口腔内异味伴有右鼻部症状。

a. 引起上述症状的原因是什么?

b. 如何进一步检查?

c. 如何治疗?

Following dental surgery this patient complains of foul-tasting debris intraorally along with right nasal symptoms.

a. What is the cause of the symptoms?

b. How would you investigate it further?

c. What is the treatment?

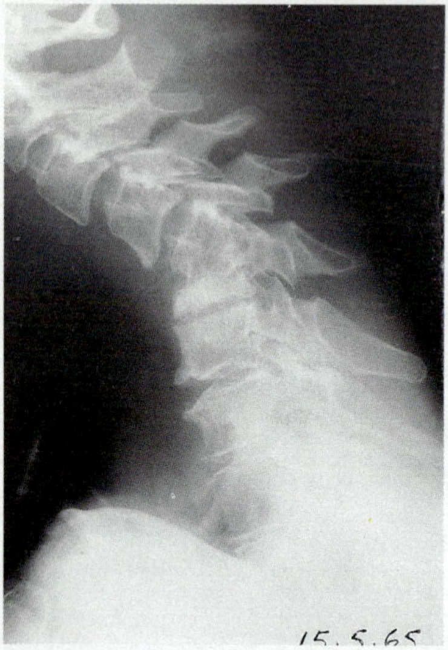

68．喉癌患者放疗术后的颈椎 X 线平片表现。

a. 该片有何异常？

b. 鉴别诊断是什么？

c. 如何治疗？

This is the cervical spine X-ray of a patient treated by radiotherapy for a laryngeal cancer.

a. What is the condition demonstrated?

b. What is the differential diagnosis?

c. How would you manage the patient?

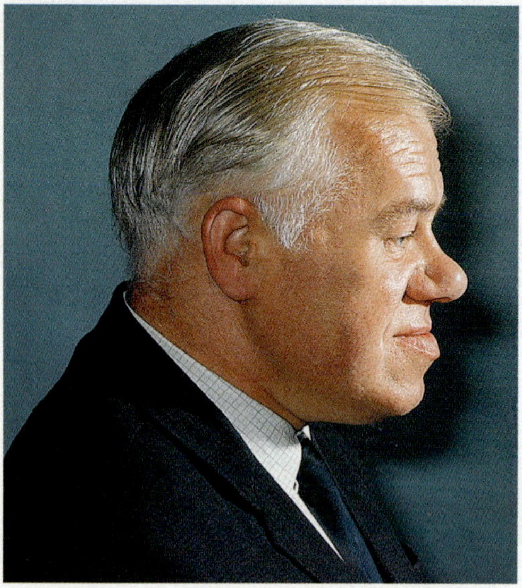

69．如图：男性患者，既往有高血压病及糖尿病。

a. 临床诊断是什么？

b. 如何确诊？

c. 可供选择的治疗方案有哪些？

This man presents with hypertension and diabetes mellitus.

a. What is the clinical diagnosis?

b. How would you confirm this?

c. What treatment options are there?

70．图为一吞咽困难患者的钡餐造影。

a. 图中可见什么表现？

b. 对该患者而言，流食与固体食物哪一种更难以下咽？

c. 在什么情况下该病可呈急性病程？

d. 治疗方案有哪些？

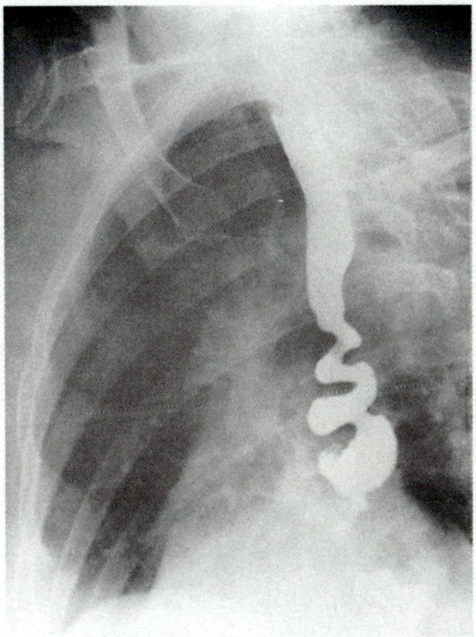

This is the barium swallow X-ray of a patient with swallowing difficulties.

a. What is the descriptive term of the condition seen?

b. Will the patient find it easier to swallow fluids or solids?

c. In what other way might it present acutely?

d. What are the treatment options?

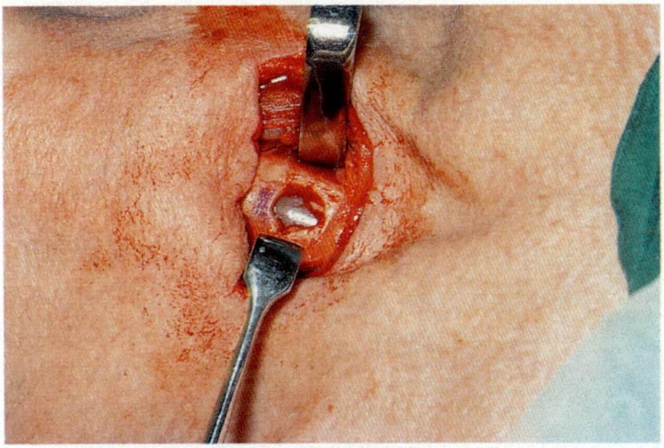

71．图为上气道梗阻患者术中所见。

a. 这是什么手术？

b. 手术适应证有哪些？

c. 对儿童患者实施该手术时应特别注意哪些问题？

This surgical procedure is being undertaken for a patient with upper airways obstruction.

a. What surgical procedure does this demonstrate?

b. What are the indications for the operation?

c. Are there specific precautions that should be undertaken when undertaking the operation in young children?

答案

1. a. 耳垂的三个小眼是人为打的耳孔。前面的小孔是先天性耳前瘘管的外口。
   b. 目前的症状说明耳前瘘管已经感染了。早期的治疗应该应用抗生素。若脓肿形成，需切开引流。待炎症控制以后，应择期切除耳前瘘管。术中应仔细切除瘘管以防复发。

   a. The three holes in her lobule are man-made ear piercings.
   b. The anterior hole is a congenital pre-auricular sinus, which has become infected. Initially treatment should be with antibiotics. Sometimes abscesses can form, which may require drainage. In the long term surgical excision should be offered, although meticulous removal is required to prevent recurrence.

2. a. 不是。棉签更容易将耵聍和脱屑推向外耳道深部，增加耳内堵塞感。
   b. 不是。鼓膜和耳道深部的上皮产生的脱屑会自然地向耳道外排出。耵聍是耳道外 1/3 的耵聍腺所分泌的，通常随上皮脱屑一同自行排出外耳道。
   c. 用棉签“清理”外耳道可能会产生一系列的问题，因此应该杜绝。棉签易将耵聍推向耳道深处而堆积在鼓膜表面。棉签也可损伤外耳道皮肤，造成外耳道炎。如果棉签插入过深，则可刺破鼓膜，甚至损伤听骨链和内耳。

   a. The use of a cotton-tipped applicator is not a good way to remove wax from the ear. The shape of the applicator makes it more likely to push wax and debris further down the external auditory canal, increasing a sensation of blockage.
   b. Wax (cerumen) does not have to be removed from the external auditory canal. The epithelium on the tympanic membrane and deep ear canal produces keratin debris, which is carried outwards by a natural active migratory process. Cerumen is produced by glandular secretion in the outer canal and is usually discharged naturally with the migrating keratin debris.
   c. Cotton-tipped applicators in the ear can cause a number of problems and should be strongly discouraged. They push the wax further down the ear canal, where it can become impacted on the

tympanic membrane. They can damage the skin of the canal and cause otitis externa. If pushed too far down the canal they can rupture the tympanic membrane and in extreme cases cause injury to the ossicles and inner ear.

3. a. 病变为耳廓皮脂腺囊肿。

   b. 手术切除为最恰当的治疗。手术可以在局麻下进行。术中应仔细清除所有上皮组织，否则囊肿可复发。

   a. The lesion is a sebaceous cyst.

   b. Surgical excision would be most appropriate. This can usually be performed under local anaesthetic. Care has to be taken to remove all of the epithelial lining, otherwise the cyst can recur.

4. a. 图片显示的是右耳“菜花状耳”，由于耳廓反复的损伤造成。耳廓的血肿使得局部软骨失去了血供，导致软骨坏死及变形。

   b. 患者患有外耳道炎，蜂窝织炎扩散至面部。最可能的病因是细菌感染。

   c. 面部蜂窝织炎应该用抗生素治疗，对严重的感染应静脉用药。对于外耳炎可采用耳部清洗，然后局部上药，通常采用抗生素和激素的联合制剂。

   a. The photograph shows a 'cauliflower ear', caused by repeated injury to the pinna. A haematoma of the pinna strips the underlying cartilage of its blood supply, with ensuing cartilage necrosis and cosmetic deformity.

   b. The patient has had otitis externa with cellulitis spreading on to the face. A bacterial infection is most likely.

   c. The facial cellulitis should be treated with antibiotics, which may have to be given intravenously for severe infections. The underlying otitis externa should be treated with aural toilet and a local medication, usually an antibiotic/steroid combination.

5. a. 诊断为先天性外耳道闭锁。

   b. 当病变为单侧时，通常不需要治疗，因为对侧耳是正常的。以往尝试重建外耳道和中耳腔的手术效果并不好，因此被摒弃了。若病变为双侧，可用骨锚式助听器。

   a. The photograph shows congenital atresia of the external auditory canal.

b. When unilateral, usually no treatment is required for hearing as the opposite ear is often normal. Attempts to surgically re-establish the external auditory canal and middle ear in the past had very poor results and have been abandoned. In bilateral cases treatment is usually insertion of a titanium implant allowing attachment of a bone-anchored hearing aid (BAHA).

6. a. 图片显示耳道深部狭窄，遮蔽了鼓膜。这种情况有时被称作“假性外耳道底”，因为看上去鼓膜似乎比正常位置浅了许多。
   b. 这种情况是由于反复发作外耳道炎或慢性外耳道炎引起。由于持续的炎症刺激，外耳道皮肤逐渐变厚，最终导致外耳道完全闭锁。
   c. 当狭窄形成时治疗变得困难。可以尝试用皮肤移植的方法来重建外耳道。也可以用激光来去除狭窄，但是常出现术后再狭窄。

   a. The photograph shows stenosis of the deep part of the external auditory canal, occluding the tympanic membrane. The condition is sometimes called a 'false fundus' as the appearance can suggest that the tympanic membrane is more laterally placed than normal.
   b. The condition arises from recurrent or chronic otitis externa. With persistent inflammation, the underlying skin becomes thickened, eventually resulting in a complete stenosis.
   c. Treatment is very difficult once stenosis has occurred. Attempts can be made to reconstruct the auditory canal with skin grafts or to remove the stenosis with a laser. However, recurrence following surgery is common.

7. a. 这是用于治疗外耳道炎的填塞物，名为Merocel™ Oto-Wick。
   b. 这种材料遇水可以膨胀。图片左侧为填塞物干燥时的状态，右侧为遇水膨胀后的状态。这种填塞物对于那些因外耳道肿胀而难以使用滴耳剂的患者来说特别有用。把填塞物塞入耳道内，然后将滴耳液滴在填塞物上，填塞物则膨胀，并且减轻耳道的肿胀。

   a. The dressing is known as a Merocel™ Oto-Wick and is used in the treatment of otitis externa.
   b. This material has the ability to expand when hydrated. On the left is the wick in its dry form, and on the right the hydrated version. This dressing is particularly useful in cases where swelling of the external auditory canal wall makes it difficult to use topical ear

drops. After insertion of the Oto-Wick the drops can be put directly on to the wick, which will then expand and lessen the canal oedema.

8. a. 图片显示的是外耳道多发的外生性骨疣。骨疣的存在可以干扰外耳道上皮自然的移行过程，导致脱屑聚集和外耳道炎。
b. 该病变被认为是“游泳者的外生性骨疣”，因该病常见于游泳者、冲浪者和潜水者。其诱因被认为是外耳道反复暴露于冷水中。
c. 对于偶尔发生的外耳道炎应该耳内清洗后滴用抗生素和激素的联合制剂。对于持续存在的外耳道炎，可以用电钻磨掉外耳道内特别突出的骨质以扩大外耳道。

a. The photograph shows multiple exostoses of the external auditory canal. These can interfere with the natural skin migration within the canal, leading to accumulation of debris and otitis externa.
b. These lesions are sometimes known as 'swimmers exostoses'. They are thought to arise from repeated exposure of the auditory canals to cold water, and are hence often found in swimmers, surfers and scuba divers.
c. Individual episodes of otitis externa should be treated with aural toilet and topical antibiotic/steroid drops. For persistent cases with marked exostosis formation the hard areas of prominent bone can be drilled down and the canal widened.

9. 右侧图片所示的方法是正确的。因为外耳道是S形的，所以应该将其拉直才能更好地看到鼓膜。这就需要将耳廓向上、向外轻拉。另外，左侧图片所示的拿耳镜的方法是不灵巧的，这样做难以精确地操控耳镜来避免损伤外耳道。

The correct method of examination is shown on the right. The external auditory canal is S-shaped and has to be straightened in order to obtain the best view of the tympanic membrane. This is achieved by gentle upward and outward traction on the pinna. In addition, in the picture on the left the otoscope is being held in an unwieldy manner in which it is more difficult to exhibit the fine control needed to avoid trauma to the external auditory canal.

10. a. 这是 Rinne 试验。
b. Rinne 试验是比较同一耳气导与骨导之间关系的试验。正常耳气导比骨导好（Rinne试验阳性）。对于中耳疾病引起的明显的传导性聋，则骨导更好（Rinne试验阴性）。若一侧耳为感音神经性聋且全聋，测骨导时，声音经颅骨传至对侧耳，得到 Rinne 试验假阴性的结果。

c. 常用频率为512Hz的音叉。低于该频率的音叉可产生声音的震动觉，而高于该频率的音叉产生的声音衰减太快而不能得到有意义的检查结果。

a. The Rinne test.

b. The Rinne test compares the responses to hearing by air and bone conduction. In a normal ear hearing by air conduction is more efficient than bone conduction and the tuning fork is heard better in air next to the ear (a positive Rinne test). In significant conductive deafness due to middle ear disease the tuning fork is heard better by bone conduction behind the ear (a negative Rinne test). In an ear with total sensorineural deafness bone conduction will be transmitted across the skull, giving a false-negative Rinne test.

c. 512Hz. Tuning forks below this frequency produce vibrotactile responses, while those above this frequency produce a sound that decays too quickly to produce a meaningful test.

11. a. 这是 Weber 试验。

b. 对于感音神经性聋的患者，音叉发出的声音主要由健耳听到。对于传导性聋的患者，由于内耳功能是正常的，音叉发出的声音主要由患耳听到。将 Rinne 试验和 Weber 试验相结合，就可以在做纯音测听之前对患者耳聋的性质作出诊断。

a. The Weber test.

b. In sensorineural deafness the tuning fork is heard predominantly in the better ear. In conductive deafness where the inner ear function is normal the tuning fork is heard predominantly in the worse ear. Using a combination of the Rinne and Weber tests the nature of deafness in a particular case can be diagnosed before confirmation by pure tone audiometry.

12. a. 这种检查被称为耳声发射（OAE）。

b. 耳声发射是由耳蜗产生的声音，可由与电脑相连接的放置于外耳道的特殊设备检测出来。在声音刺激下若能出现耳声发射，则证明耳蜗功能正常。全世界都用新生儿听力筛查来早期发现耳聋。耳聋发现得越早，就可以越及时地进行听力康复。这样患儿就有机会最大限度地发展言语和语言的能力。

a. Testing for evoked otoacoustic emissions (OAE), sometimes known as 'cochlear echoes'.

b. Otoacoustic emissions are sounds produced by the cochlea, which can be detected by sophisticated equipment placed in the external ear canal and linked to a computer. The presence of an evoked otoacoustic emission in response to a sound stimulus is a good indicator of normal cochlear function. Universal neonatal hearing screening is used to detect deafness at an early stage. The earlier significant deafness is detected the earlier appropriate rehabilitation can be given. In this way the chances of developing optimum speech and language development can be maximized.

13. a. 他做了安装骨锚式助听器（BAHA）的手术。图片显示的是BAHA 的固定装置。在患者耳后的颅骨上已经安装了螺钉。螺钉表面的皮肤和皮下组织被去除，代之以没有毛发的移植皮片。

b. BAHA用于无法在外耳道佩戴常规助听器的患者。如先天性外耳道闭锁，慢性外耳道炎所致的反复耳流脓，或者慢性中耳炎。声波可以直接通过 BAHA 以骨传导的方式传至耳蜗。

a. The photograph shows an abutment for a bone-anchored hearing aid (BAHA). A screw fixture has been inserted into the skull behind the ear. The overlying skin and subcutaneous tissue has been removed and replaced with a non-hairy skin graft.

b. BAHAs are used in people who cannot wear a conventional hearing aid in the external ear canal. This may be because of congenital atresia of the canals, recurrent discharge due to chronic otitis externa, or chronic otitis media. Sound impulses are conducted directly via the BAHA to the cochlea by bone conduction.

14. a. 若长时间暴露于强声中，主要的危害是导致噪声性聋。耳聋的程度取决于噪声的强度、暴露的时间及个体的易感性。音乐家若站在扬声器附近就易患噪声性聋。

b. 症状是隐匿的、缓慢出现的。起初患者可能会出现耳聋和耳鸣，但是是可逆的（暂时性阈移）。如反复暴露于噪声中，则出现永久性的耳聋和耳鸣。

c. 一旦出现永久性耳聋，听力是不可能恢复的。严重的病例可使用助听器。以后尽可能少地接触噪声是非常重要的。

a. The principal risk is of noise-induced deafness with exposure over a prolonged period of time. The degree of deafness in an individual depends on the loudness of the noise, duration of exposure and individual susceptibility. Musicians are at risk when positioned close to loudspeakers.

b. The symptoms are insidious. At first there maybe deafness and tinnitus, which initially is reversible (temporary threshold shift). After repeated exposure permanent deafness and tinnitus may occur.

c. Once permanent deafness has occurred the hearing cannot be restored. In severe cases a hearing aid maybe useful. Minimization of future noise exposure is vital.

15. a. 这是 Epley 耳石复位法。用于治疗良性阵发性位置性眩晕(BPPV)。

b. BPPV 被认为是耳石脱落至前庭迷路，然后通常进入后半规管，刺激半规管壶腹所致。Epley 手法的目的是通过移动头位，使耳石从后半规管出来进入前庭，而不再刺激壶腹产生症状。

a. An Epley particle-repositioning manoeuvre, used in the treatment of benign paroxysmal positional vertigo (BPPV).

b. It is thought that BPPV is due to debris collecting in the vestibular labyrinth, usually the posterior semicircular canal, and stimulation of the canal ampulla. The aim of the Epley manoeuvre is to move the head in order to encourage the debris to flow away from the posterior canal into the vestibule of the inner ear, where it no longer causes a problem.

16. a. 监测的是面神经的功能。

b. 面神经自脑干发出，穿经颞骨，在腮腺内分成数支。因此在颞骨颅底手术、乳突切除术和腮腺切除术中有损伤面神经的可能性；另外，下颌下腺手术有可能损伤面神经的下颌缘支，面神经功能监测就是应用于上述这些手术当中。

c. 面神经监测仪检测的是由于刺激面神经时面肌产生的电生理活动。这种电生理活动可被麻醉过程中使用的神经肌肉阻断剂所阻断。因此使用面神经监测仪时应注意神经肌肉阻断剂的应用。

a. The function of the facial nerve.

b. The facial nerve travels from the brainstem through the temporal bone to branch in the parotid gland. The nerve is hence at risk during temporal bone skull base surgery, mastoidectomy and parotidectomy, and is monitored during these operations. The marginal mandibular branch of the facial nerve is also at risk during surgery of the submandibular salivary gland.

c. The facial nerve monitor detects electrical activity in the facial muscles in response to manipulation of the facial nerve. This activity is abolished by neuromuscular blocking agents used to produce paralysis during anaesthesia. These drugs must therefore be used with caution during facial nerve monitoring.

17. a. 这个患者做的是开放式的乳突根治术及耳道成型术以扩大外耳道。因此术后外耳道异常地宽大。而常规的助听器难以适合这样宽大的外耳道。另外，乳突根治术后术腔所产生的分泌物也妨碍了常规助听器的使用。

b. 这个患者佩戴的是骨锚式助听器(BAHA)，通过钛螺钉固定在颅骨上。

a. The clue is in the size of the external auditory canal, which is abnormally large. The patient has had an open cavity mastoidectomy performed which includes a meatoplasty to widen the ear canal. With a very wide ear canal obtaining the close fit required for a hearing aid to work may be a problem. In addition, some mastoidectomy cavities discharge, which would also hinder hearing aid use.

b. The patient is wearing a bone-anchored hearing aid (BAHA) attached to a titanium fixture inserted into the bone of the skull.

18. a. 诊断是中耳积液，可见液平面。

b. 可能的潜在病变是鼻咽癌继发颈淋巴结转移。由于癌肿阻塞咽鼓管口而造成中耳积液。

c. 鼻咽癌常见于华人。EB 病毒感染被认为是致病原因。

d. 可采用中耳置管来治疗中耳积液。需进行鼻咽部活检来确诊鼻咽癌。治疗采用放疗联合化疗，对于颈部残留病变可采用手术切除。

a. A serous effusion in the middle ear with a fluid level.

b. Nasopharyngeal carcinoma with secondary spread to the cervical lymph nodes. The middle ear effusion is caused by obstruction of the Eustachian tube.

c. Nasopharyngeal carcinoma is common in those of Chinese origin. Epstein-Barr virus has been implicated in the aetiology.

d. The middle ear effusion can be treated with ventilation tube insertion. A biopsy needs to be taken of the nasopharynx to confirm the diagnosis of carcinoma. Treatment is then usually a combination of radiotherapy and cytotoxic chemotherapy, with surgery for residual neck disease.

19. a. 图片显示鼓膜紧张部前半部分以及上鼓室区域的鼓膜内陷。由于内陷的鼓膜非常薄，常被误认为是穿孔。仔细观察可以辨别非常薄的鼓膜。另外在前方可能有积液。

b. 这种现象是由于咽鼓管功能不良导致的。在患者幼年的时候可能多次接受过中耳置管的治疗。

c. 目前的治疗取决于患者的临床症状。如果耳聋是中度的且对侧耳正常，则无需治疗。如果耳聋严重，影响语言交流，则可尝试戴助听器。一些医生提倡重建术，因为内陷的鼓膜可以发展为胆脂瘤。

a. The photograph shows retraction of the tympanic membrane in the anterior part of the pars tensa and the superior attic regions. This type of retraction where the drum is very thin is often mistaken for a perforation. Careful inspection, however, usually reveals the thin membrane. In addition there is a possible effusion seen behind the drum anteriorly.

b. This appearance is the result of poor Eustachian tube function. In earlier childhood repeated insertions of ventilation tubes (grommets) may have been undertaken.

c. Current management depends on the symptoms. If the degree of deafness is mild and the opposite ear is normal no treatment is required. If deafness is a problem then a hearing aid could be contemplated. Some surgeons would advocate reconstructive surgery, arguing that the retraction of the drum can subsequently develop into cholesteatoma.

20. a. 做的是鼓膜置管术，即将鼓膜通气管置入鼓膜。

b. 中耳积液（胶耳）患者应当行置管术。

c. 中耳积液通常引起传导性耳聋，影响患儿的学习及言语发育。除中耳置管外，还可以佩戴助听器。还有一些人建议用经鼻咽鼓管吹张的办法来改善咽鼓管的通气功能。另外，中耳置管的同时应做腺样体切除术以减少复发率。

d. 可以游泳。在游泳池和海水中游泳时没必要用耳塞，因为表面张力作用可以防止水进入中耳。肥皂水表面张力小且有刺激性。因此耳鼻喉科医生通常建议患者洗头和淋浴时用浸有石油凝胶的棉球堵住耳朵。

a. Insertion of a ventilation tube or grommet in the tympanic membrane.

b. Ventilation tubes are inserted for otitis media with effusion (OME/glue ear).

c. OME usually presents with conductive deafness. Children can have problems at school and poor speech development. One alternative to ventilation tubes is the use of hearing aids. Also, some advocate the use of an Otovent - this is basically a nasal balloon-blowing device aimed to improve Eustachian tube ventilation. In addition adenoidectomy performed at the same time as ventilation tube insertion can reduce the recurrence rate.

d. The child can swim. There is no need for earplugs with swimming pool water and sea water, as the surface tension effect prevents water from entering the middle ear. Soapy water lowers surface tension and is irritant. For this reason ENT surgeons usually recommend the use of cotton wool with petroleum jelly to plug the ears during shampooing and showering.

21. a. 图片显示中耳置管已被自然地排出。在鼓膜前下部可见残留的穿孔，此处是原来置管的位置。

b. 置管排出后残留的穿孔95%会自行愈合。排出的置管会随着上皮移行自然地从外耳道内排出。最后置管会与耵聍一起被排出外耳道。

a. The photograph shows a ventilation tube (grommet) that has been naturally extruded from the tympanic membrane. There is a residual perforation in the anterior part of the drum, where the tube was originally positioned.

b. Following extrusion of ventilation tubes the residual perforation heals spontaneously in about 95% of cases. The extruding tube will be carried along the external auditory canal by the natural process of epithelial migration. Eventually the tube will become mixed with the wax in the outer part of the canal and usually fall out of the ear.

22. a. 图片显示在鼓膜的前部可见肉芽，这种情况被称为“肉芽性鼓膜炎”。有肉芽的区域表示局部有感染。该病的发病和病因常常是隐匿的。

b. 最常见的症状是耳流脓，可以是持续性的或间歇性的。

c. 局部使用抗生素 / 激素滴耳剂或膏剂对多数病例有效。局部用硝酸银烧灼也是有效的。一些病例非常难治。在某些非常严重的病例，可以切除长有肉芽的鼓膜，然后行鼓膜成形术。

a. The photograph shows a granular area in the anterior part of the tympanic membrane - a condition known as 'granular myringitis'. The area represents localized infection, the onset and aetiology of which is often obscure.

b. The most common symptom is purulent discharge from the ear, which may be persistent or intermittent.

c. Many cases respond to local treatment with topical antibiotic/ steroid drops or ointment. The use of local chemical cautery with silver nitrate can also be successful. Some cases are very resistant to treatment. In the most severe cases excision of the affected segment and grafting as in a myringoplasty operation may be required.

23. a. 鼓膜后部的外伤性鼓膜穿孔。症状取决于外伤的程度。多数患者表现为轻度的耳聋、耳鸣和耳内流出血性分泌物。如果伤及听骨链，耳聋会更严重。最严重的是伤及内耳，外淋巴液从卵圆窗或圆窗漏出，伴感音神经性聋和眩晕。

b. 多数外伤性鼓膜穿孔在数周内会自行愈合。保持耳内干燥是非常重要的。没必要服用抗生素来预防。少数患者穿孔未自行愈合，需行鼓膜成形术。

a. Traumatic perforation of the posterior part of the tympanic membrane. The symptoms depend on the degree of trauma. Most cases present with mild deafness, tinnitus and blood-stained discharge from the ear. If the ossicular chain is damaged the deafness will be more severe. In the most severe cases the inner ear can be traumatized, with leak of perilymph from the oval or round windows accompanied by sensorineural deafness and vertigo.

b. Most traumatic tympanic membrane perforations heal spontaneously within a few weeks. It is important to keep the ear dry. Antibiotic prophylaxis is not necessary. For the uncommon case in which healing does not occur, surgical repair with a myringoplasty operation may be required.

24. a. 正在流脓的鼓膜中央型穿孔。
    b. 最可能的致病菌是革兰阴性菌，如假单胞菌和变形杆菌。
    c. 最有效的治疗是抗生素 / 激素滴耳液。许多抗生素滴耳液含有氨基糖苷类药物， 如庆大霉素，有一定的内耳毒性。与持续流脓对内耳的毒性相比，这些抗生素滴耳液的毒性是轻微的。也可以用含有喹诺酮类药物的滴耳液，如氧氟沙星。口服广谱抗生素通常无效。如果穿孔持续存在，最终需行鼓膜成形术。

    a. A discharging central perforation.
    b. The most common infective agents are Gram-negative organisms such as *Pseudomonas* spp. and *Proteus* spp.
    c. The most effective treatment is antibiotic/steroid ear drops. Most antibiotic ear-drop preparations contain aminoglycosides such as gentamicin and present a small risk of inner ear ototoxicity. This small risk, however, is outweighed by the risk to the inner ear of continued purulent infection. An alternative is to use drops containing quinolone preparations such as ofloxacin. Broad-spectrum oral antibiotics are usually ineffective. If the perforation persists, surgical closure with a myringoplasty operation may eventually be necessary.

25. a. 自乳突气房至表面皮肤的耳后瘘管，伴有脓肿形成。
    b. 最可能的病变是胆脂瘤。在发展中国家，耳鼻喉专科服务很缺乏，导致慢性中耳疾病发展至严重的程度。胆脂瘤所引起的危及生命的颅内并发症在这些国家也更为常见。

    a. A postauricular fistula between the mastoid air cells and the skin, with abscess formation.
    b. Cholesteatoma. In developing countries where access to specialized ENT care is poor, chronic middle ear disease often presents at a late stage. Life-threatening intracranial complications of cholesteatoma are also more common.

26. a. 这张图片显示在鼓膜紧张部后上部分可见一白色结构。通过这一表现诊断可能为胆脂瘤、鼓室硬化症或人工听小骨。事实上，这个白色结构是羟基磷灰石制成的人工听小骨。
    b. 这名患者做的是听骨链成形术。这种手术旨在重建中耳听骨链的连续性，从而重建听力。听骨链连续性的破坏常常由于既往中耳感染且常由胆脂瘤引起。最常见的听骨链破坏是砧骨长脚的缺失，在这种情况下人工听小骨可以置于镫骨头和鼓膜或锤骨之间。若镫骨足弓缺失，则需将人工听小骨置于镫骨底板和鼓膜之间，但是效果往往不理想。

a. The photograph shows a white structure in the posterior-superior part of the pars tensa of the tympanic membrane. Diagnostic possibilities characterized by their white appearance are cholesteatoma, tympanosclerosis and artificial replacement ossicles. In fact this particular white structure is a replacement ossicle made from synthetic hydroxyapatite.

b. The patient has hence undergone an ossiculoplasty operation. These operations are designed to restore the continuity of the middle ear ossicular chain and hence restore hearing. Ossicular discontinuity usually arises as a result of previous middle ear infection and is often associated with cholesteatoma. The commonest defect is loss of the long process of the incus, in which case a prosthesis can be inserted between the stapes head and drum or malleus. Loss of the stapes arch requires a prosthesis to be inserted between the stapes footplate and the drum, the results of which are often disappointing.

27. a. 诊断是鼓膜中央型的干穿孔。

b. 传导性聋。

c. (1) 穿孔的大小和位置。穿孔越大听力越差——鼓膜后部的穿孔可造成更严重的耳聋，因为穿孔位于圆窗和卵圆窗的表面。

(2) 听骨链中断——砧骨长脚或镫骨足弓的破坏可造成严重的耳聋。

(3) 活动性耳流脓——流脓的耳比干耳更聋。

(4) 鼓室硬化症可造成听骨链固定和残余鼓膜活动障碍。

a. A dry central perforation of the tympanic membrane.

b. Conductive deafness.

c. (1) Size and position of the perforation. The larger the perforation the greater the deafness - posterior perforations are associated with greater deafness because they lie over the round and oval windows.

(2) Associated ossicular discontinuity - erosion of the incus long process or the stapes arch are associated with greater deafness.

(3) Active discharge - a wet ear is deafer than a dry ear.

(4) Tympanosclerosis can cause fixation of the ossicles and immobility of the tympanic membrane remnant.

28. a. 鼓膜松弛部或上鼓室区域可见胆脂瘤。
b. 胆脂瘤可以破坏骨质。在中耳和乳突区域胆脂瘤可以造成面神经麻痹，并破坏内耳，引起化脓性迷路炎。胆脂瘤也可以引起颅内并发症，如脑膜炎、颅内脓肿和乙状窦血栓。
c. 需行乳突切除手术。有几种不同的方式，目的都是清除胆脂瘤和保持患耳干燥、安全。

a. Cholesteatoma in the pars flaccida or attic region of the tympanic membrane.
b. Cholesteatoma has the ability to erode bone. In the middle ear and mastoid this can result in facial nerve paralysis and erosion into the inner ear, causing suppurative labyrinthitis. Spread outside the temporal bone can cause intracranial complications such as meningitis, intracranial abscess and lateral sinus thrombosis.
c. A mastoidectomy operation. There are various techniques, which all aim to remove the cholesteatoma and restore a dry, safe ear.

29. a. 右耳比左耳突出，外观尚正常。
b. 鉴别诊断包括先天性的招风耳、急性乳突炎和急性外耳道炎伴耳后淋巴结肿大。针对这个特殊病例，诊断为急性外耳道炎。
c. 通过病史和查体常能作出诊断。急性乳突炎和外耳道炎常有耳痛，可能有耳流脓和耳聋。急性外耳道炎的患者牵拉耳廓时会疼痛。对于难以诊断的病例，尤其需行乳突凿开术时，需做颞骨 CT。

a. The right ear is more prominent than the left. The appearance is otherwise normal.
b. The differential diagnosis includes a congenitally prominent ear, acute mastoiditis and acute otitis externa with postaural lymph nodes. In this particular case the diagnosis was acute otitis externa.
c. History and examination will usually reveal the diagnosis. In acute mastoiditis and otitis externa there will be earache with possibly discharge and deafness. In acute otitis externa traction on the pinna will be painful. In some cases where the diagnosis is difficult a CT scan of the temporal bone may be required, particularly where a cortical mastoidectomy may be required.

30. a. 图片显示耳道深部的脓液。在鼓膜后上象限与耳道的交界处（即鼓环处）可见一红色的肉芽组织，这一表现提示在中耳腔的后部可能有胆脂瘤，也可能向后方侵入乳突。
b. 他很有可能患有急性乳突炎。
c. 如果已经有耳后脓肿则需手术切开引流。耳后蜂窝织炎不伴脓肿形成则需静脉抗生素治疗。对于胆脂瘤需行乳突切除术。

a. The photograph shows discharge in the deep ear canal. There is reddish granulation tissue at the junction of the ear canal and the tympanic membrane (tympanic annulus) in the posterior-superior part. The appearance is suggestive of underlying cholesteatoma in the posterior marginal region of the middle ear, with possible spread into the mastoid posteriorly.
b. It is likely that acute mastoiditis has arisen.
c. If a postauricular abscess is present surgical drainage is needed. Postaural cellulitis without abscess may respond to intravenous antibiotics. Underlying cholesteatoma will require mastoidectomy surgery.

31. a. 左耳鼓膜后方的干穿孔。
b. 在图片左部可以看到锤骨柄。穿孔位于砧镫关节的表面。横跨穿孔的白色结构是镫骨肌腱。

a. A dry posterior perforation of the left tympanic membrane.
b. In the left of the picture the handle of the malleus can be seen. The perforation itself overlies the incudo-stapedial joint. The white structure passing horizontally across the perforation is the tendon of the stapedius muscle.

32. a. 类固醇激素鼻喷剂。该例患者使用的药物是倍他米松。
b. 目的是使药物到达鼻腔上部和筛窦区域。
c. 鼻息肉病。
d. 最主要的危险是类固醇激素的全身吸收和肾上腺功能的抑制。由于倍他米松鼻喷剂的这种副作用，一次连续用药一般限制在 6 周内。

a. A nasal drop preparation containing a steroid, in this case betamethasone.
b. In order to reach the upper parts of the nasal cavity and ethmoidal regions.
c. Nasal polyposis.

d. The main danger is systemic absorption of steroid medication and adrenal suppression. This is a particular risk of intranasal betamethasone treatment, which as a result is limited to a maximum of 6 weeks at a time.

33. a. 照片显示左眼向下移位。由于左眼视轴不正常，导致了复视。

b. CT显示筛窦和额窦模糊。另外，在左侧额窦的外侧可见囊肿形成，这是由于额窦引流口阻塞所形成的黏液囊肿。尽管黏液囊肿是良性病变，但它可使周围骨质压迫吸收。该例患者眶顶的骨质已经压迫吸收，并且挤压眼球向下移位引起复视。

a. The photograph shows that the left eye is at a lower horizontal level than the right. The axis of vision for the left eye is abnormal, hence the diplopia.

b. The CT scan shows opacity of the ethmoid and frontal sinuses. In addition there is a cystic collection in the lateral part of the left frontal sinus, known as a mucocele, caused by obstruction to frontal sinus outflow. Although the mucocele is a benign condition, pressure erosion of adjacent bone can occur. In this case the bone forming the roof of the orbit has been eroded, with downward displacement of the globe, and resulting diplopia.

34. a. 鼻堵、脓涕症状提示为慢性鼻窦炎。额窦的慢性感染偶可通过皮肤破溃，形成瘘管。由鼻窦的慢性感染侵蚀前颅底骨引起颅内并发症如脑膜炎和颅内脓肿的情况更少见。

b. 首先检查鼻腔确定为鼻窦感染，然后进行鼻窦 CT 扫描确定病变范围和除外颅内并发症。该例患者应手术重建鼻窦引流，同时切除瘘管。

a. The symptoms of nasal stuffiness and purulent nasal discharge are suggestive of chronic sinus infection. Occasionally chronic infection of the frontal sinus can erode through the skin, resulting in a cutaneous fistula. Chronic sinus infections can also on rare occasions erode the bone protecting the anterior cranial fossa and present with intracranial complications such as meningitis and intracerebral abscess.

b. The nasal cavity should be examined to look for evidence of sinus infection. A CT scan should be obtained to define the extent of sinus disease and exclude intracranial complications. In this case surgery will probably be needed in order to re-establish sinus drainage, and also to remove the fistula.

35. a. Kaposi 肉瘤。

b. 大多数 Kaposi 肉瘤的皮肤病变是无症状的，因此无须治疗。如果影响美观，可手术切除。放疗和化疗均对Kaposi肉瘤有效，用于治疗HIV感染的抗逆转录病毒制剂对Kaposi肉瘤也有效。

a. Kaposi's sarcoma.

b. Most Kaposi's sarcoma lesions are asymptomatic and no treatment may be required. If cosmetically unsightly the lesions may be excised. Kaposi's sarcoma will also respond to radiotherapy or chemotherapy. Treatment of the underlying HIV infection with anti-retroviral agents will also produce resolution of Kaposi's sarcoma.

36. a. 前方为四方软骨，后为犁骨，上为筛骨垂直板。

b. 嗅丝。嗅黏膜位于鼻腔顶，是由感受嗅觉的特殊上皮组成。嗅素通过鼻腔刺激嗅上皮的感受器，通过嗅丝穿过筛板上的筛孔组成嗅神经（第一脑神经），经前颅底窝到达嗅皮质产生嗅觉。

a. Quadrilateral cartilage anteriorly, vomer bone posteriorly and the perpendicular plate of the ethmoid bone superiorly.

b. Olfactory filaments. The olfactory mucosa is specialized epithelium lying in the roof of the nasal cavity. The epithelium mediates the sense of smell. Odours passing into the nose stimulate receptors in the olfactory epithelium. Olfactory filaments then pass through small holes in the cribriform plate part of the ethmoid bone. These filaments then combine to form the olfactory nerves (the first cranial nerves), which run in the floor of the anterior cranial fossa into the olfactory cortex.

37. a. 鼻咽部恶性肿瘤。常见的肿瘤是鳞癌和淋巴瘤。鼻咽癌在东南亚华人中最常见，它是最具有流行病学特点的恶性肿瘤之一。常被认为与 EB 病毒感染有关。

b. 颈部肿块高度怀疑为颈淋巴结转移，诊断可通过针吸进行细胞学检查。鼻咽部恶性肿瘤可阻塞咽鼓管，引起中耳渗液，导致耳聋。

a. A malignant tumour of the nasopharynx. The two common tumours are squamous carcinoma and lymphoma. Nasopharyngeal carcinoma is particularly common in the Chinese community in south east Asia, where it is one of the most prevalent malignant diseases. It is thought to be related to Epstein-Barr virus infection.

b. The neck lump would be highly suspicious of a metastatic lymph node. Diagnosis could be confirmed by fine-needle aspiration for cytology. Blockage of the Eustachian tube by a nasopharyngeal malignancy causes deafness by production of a middle ear effusion.

38. a. 照片显示单侧鼻息肉，且息肉已使右鼻腔扩大，近期还发生过鼻出血。

b. 应与单侧息肉样新生物鉴别。最常见的新生物是良性内翻性乳突状瘤。恶性肿瘤较少见且预后较差，如恶性唾液腺肿瘤、黑色素瘤、鳞癌和嗅神经母细胞瘤。在硬木材工业区工作的工人鼻腔鼻窦囊性腺癌的发病率较高。该病例实际上是双侧单纯性鼻息肉，右侧较左侧严重。

c. 恶性肿瘤的症状包括涕中带血、面部肿胀、复视、牙齿松动和中耳积液引起的耳聋。

a. The photograph shows a unilateral nasal polyp. The polyp has caused some expansion of the right nasal cavity. There is evidence of recent bleeding.

b. With unilateral nasal polyps neoplasia must be suspected. The commonest nasal neoplasm is the benign inverted papilloma. Malignant nasal neoplasms are rare but often have a poor prognosis. Examples are malignant salivary gland tumours, melanoma, squamous carcinoma and olfactory neuroblastoma. Sinonasal adenocarcinoma is more common in workers employed in the hardwood industry. In this particular case the other possibility is that the patient actually has bilateral simple polyps, with the right side being more severely affected.

c. Symptoms suggestive of malignancy include blood-stained nasal discharge, facial swelling, diplopia, loose teeth and deafness due to middle ear effusion.

39. a. 照片显示黏液性分泌物经鼻腔流入鼻咽。“卡他”症状是一种病态现象，大多数人认为是分泌的黏液过多而经后鼻孔滴漏流入鼻咽部。“卡他”也被称为后鼻滴漏。正常鼻腔通过鼻黏膜内的腺体和杯状细胞分泌大量黏液。这些黏液是清亮的，随纤毛运动进入鼻咽。当鼻腔或鼻窦感染时，鼻分泌物就变稠呈脓性。

b. 正常清亮的鼻分泌物是生理性的，很难消除。但如果是脓性分泌物应考虑鼻 - 鼻窦炎。治疗要根据病史和鼻内镜检查所见决定治疗方案。

a. The photograph shows a stream of mucus passing from the nasal cavity into the nasopharynx. The symptom of 'catarrh' is ill-defined - most people describe excess mucus in the nasopharynx. Catarrh is also known as postnasal discharge (PND). The nasal cavity normally produces a large quantity of mucus from glands and goblet cells within the nasal lining. This mucus is carried towards the nasopharynx by the action of cilia, and is normally clear fluid. When there is infection in the nose or sinuses the nasal secretions can become thick and purulent.

b. The normal clear nasal secretions are physiological and difficult to abolish. If there is purulent secretion rhinosinusitis would have to be suspected and treated depending on the history and endoscopic findings.

40. a. 是由于鼻中隔前部偏曲，也称鼻小柱偏曲引起的鼻堵。此区的鼻中隔是由软骨组成，多因外伤致偏曲。大多数患者的病史较长，常从儿童开始，随着面部的发育而逐渐加重。

b. 如果鼻堵影响正常生活，就应行鼻中隔矫正术。手术时要将软骨与骨连接处松动，重新复位。由于软骨有“记忆”功能，常使手术失败，这是由于复位的软骨又回到了术前的位置。但如果切除鼻中隔前方的软骨，有可能会发生鼻尖塌陷影响外观。

a. The photograph shows a deviation of the anterior part of the nasal septum, also known as the columella. This part of the septum is composed of cartilage. The deviation may have resulted from a previous nasal injury. In many cases deviation takes place over many years, starting in childhood and slowly increasing with facial growth.

b. If the nasal blockage is troublesome a corrective surgical procedure called a septoplasty could be performed. In this procedure the cartilage is mobilized from its bony attachments and repositioned. Because cartilage has a 'memory' these operations are sometimes unsuccessful as the repositioned cartilage adopts its former position. If anterior septal cartilage is removed cosmetic nasal deformity with nasal collapse may occur.

41. a. 图为舌弥漫性肿胀，充满口腔。如果起病急，可能为急性变态反应或血管性水肿（补体系统异常）。
b. 紧急处理是保持呼吸道通畅，如果鼻腔通畅可插入鼻咽通气管。如发生危及生命的上呼吸道阻塞，应紧急经鼻气管插管或行气管造口术。
c. 急诊处理的药物治疗是应用 1：1000 的肾上腺素和皮质类固醇激素，如地塞米松静脉点滴或肌肉注射。另外，也可用氯苯那敏等抗组胺类药物。

a. The photograph shows a diffusely swollen tongue that appears to be filling the oral cavity. The acute onset suggests either an acute allergic reaction or an episode of angio-oedema (a disorder of the complement system).
b. The immediate concern is to secure the airway. If the nasal cavity is patent a nasopharyngeal airway could be inserted. With life-threatening severe upper airway obstruction naso-tracheal intubation or emergency tracheostomy may be needed.
c. In the acute situation 1:1000 adrenaline (epinephrine) and a corticosteroid such as dexamethasone would be useful, given by intravenous or intramuscular injection. In addition an antihistamine preparation such as chlorphenamine (chlorpheniramine) could also be given.

42. a. 视神经走行于蝶窦外侧壁，损伤视神经可引起失明。
b. 筛窦比邻前颅底，如损伤前颅底可导致脑脊液漏；损伤颈内动脉引起的严重出血是极少见的。以上并发症虽然少见，但应高度重视。

a. The optic nerve running in the lateral part of the sphenoid sinus. Damage to the optic nerve can cause blindness.
b. The ethmoid sinuses are also close to the anterior skull base, which if damaged can result in a leak of cerebrospinal fluid. Severe bleeding can rarely occur as a result of damage to the interior carotid artery. These complications, while rare, are well recognized.

43. a. CT显示眶底板骨质缺损，部分眶内容物突入上颌窦内。这种外伤称“击出性骨折”。
b. 这种外伤引起复视的原因有两种：一是眶内容物下陷引起视轴成线错位，它可通过眶底假体修复来纠正；二是眼肌嵌顿，需行眶探查术直接修复。

a. The CT scan shows a defect in the bone of the orbital floor with partial prolapse of the orbital contents into the maxillary antrum. This injury is known as a 'blowout' fracture of the orbit.
b. Double vision can occur with this injury for two reasons. First, the downward prolapse of the orbital contents may cause malalignment of the orbital axis, which could be corrected by prosthetic repair of the orbital floor. Second, some of the orbital muscles may have become entrapped, requiring direct repair via an orbital exploration.

44. a. 眶蜂窝织炎。
b. 眶周和眶组织蜂窝织炎可因局部眶内感染引起，也可因邻近鼻窦感染的扩散引起。
c. 通常短期静脉应用抗生素。严重病例，CT显示是继发于鼻窦炎者应行鼻窦手术进行引流。如果治疗不及时，部分患者可发展成眶内脓肿，造成永久性失明。

a. Orbital cellulitis.
b. Cellulitis of the periorbital and orbital tissues can either result from local orbital infection or spread from the neighbouring sinuses.
c. Usually the condition responds to a short course of intravenous antibiotics. In severe cases a CT scan may reveal underlying sinusitis, which may have to be surgically drained. Left untreated, some cases may progress to orbital abscess formation, with a risk of permanent blindness.

45. a. 遗传性出血性毛细血管扩张症。
b. 常染色体显性遗传。
c. 该病鼻出血常较严重，需反复住院治疗。一般电灼或鼻腔填塞无明显效果，其他多种治疗方法如激光治疗、鼻中隔皮肤移植、鼻孔封闭等也无显著疗效。

a. Hereditary haemorrhagic telangiectasia (Osler-Weber-Rendu syndrome).
b. Autosomal dominant.
c. These patients can often suffer with severe epistaxis requiring repeated hospital admission. The usual measures of nasal cautery and packing are often not effective. Many alternative types of treatment such as laser therapy, skin grafting of the nasal septum and surgical closure of the nostrils (Young's procedure) have been

performed, but with limited success.

46. a. 泪囊的黏脓囊肿。通过皮肤破溃形成窦道流脓。形成的原因是鼻腔外侧壁远端鼻泪管阻塞，泪液不能从泪囊流入鼻腔的下鼻道。泪囊感染称泪囊炎。
    b. 通过泪囊鼻腔吻合术将泪道系统的泪液引流至鼻腔。在近中鼻甲处鼻腔外侧壁的骨质做一骨窗，使泪囊在鼻腔内造一大瘘孔。该手术有两种途径，鼻外手术或鼻内镜下经鼻手术。

    a. Muco-pyocele of the lacrimal sac, which has discharged through the skin to form a sinus. The underlying cause is blockage of the distal nasolacrimal duct in the lateral wall of the nasal cavity. Tears are not able to flow normally through the lacrimal sac into the inferior meatus of the nasal cavity. Infection of the lacrimal sac then occurs, known as dacryocystitis.
    b. The treatment is to ensure drainage of the lacrimal system into the nasal cavity by an operation known as a dacryocystorhinostomy or DCR. The bone of the upper lateral nasal wall is removed, creating a large ostium from the lacrimal sac into the nasal cavity near the middle turbinate. This procedure can be performed through an external incision or endoscopically through the nose.

47. a. 先天性鳃裂瘘管。它是由于胎儿发育过程中，鳃弓和鳃裂系统发育异常所致。鳃弓和鳃裂与头颈部大多数结构的发育有关。
    b. 该例患儿瘘管已形成，需手术切除瘘管。由于瘘管常走行于颈部深层，而典型的瘘管还与腭扁桃体附近的咽部相通，故手术彻底切除瘘管常较困难。

    a. Congenital branchial fistula. These result from failure of complete development of the branchial arch and cleft system in utero. This system is responsible for the development of most of the structures of the head and neck.
    b. This particular patient opted to leave the lesion alone. The lesion can be excised, although the surgery is often difficult as the internal track of the fistula can pass deeply into the neck and classically has a communication with the pharynx near the palatine tonsil.

48. a. 鼻乳头状瘤。
    b. 与人乳头状瘤病毒感染有关。
    c. 不是。

d. 手术切除，有复发倾向。

a. A nasal papilloma (wart).
b. Human papilloma virus (HPV).
c. No.
d. Surgical excision, although these lesions have a tendency to recur.

49. a. 有两种可能的疾病：鳞状细胞癌和基底细胞癌。基底细胞癌生长较缓慢，鳞状细胞癌可扩散至区域淋巴结。
b. 手术或放射治疗。手术切除后常需要皮瓣或假体修复缺损。

a. The two main diagnostic possibilities are squamous and basal cell carcinoma. Basal cell carcinoma tends to be slower growing. Squamous cell carcinoma can spread to regional lymph nodes.
b. Surgery or radiotherapy. Surgical treatment will require skin flap or prosthetic repair of any resulting defect.

50. a. 鼻腔下鼻甲黏膜肿胀，表面附黏液性分泌物。
b. 花粉过敏（草或树）。其他可能的变应原有屋尘螨或动物皮屑，这些变应原可引起常年变应性症状。
c. 花粉过敏的药物治疗包括：抗组胺药、鼻内类固醇激素喷雾剂、色甘酸钠喷雾剂（肥大细胞稳定剂）。

a. The inferior turbinate in the nasal cavity. The lining mucosa is swollen, with clear mucus present.
b. Allergy to pollen (grass or tree). Other possible allergens are house dust mite or animal fur, although these would tend to cause year-round (perennial) symptoms.
c. Medications used for pollen allergy include antihistamines, nasal steroid sprays and disodium chromoglycate spray (mast cell stabilizer).

51. a. 全喉切除标本，已经喉前壁裂开。标本中可见大面积黏膜溃疡，提示鳞状细胞癌。
b. 喉癌大多发生于长期吸烟的患者，特别是同时有长期饮酒史的人群。
c. 早期喉癌病变常局限于喉内。进展期病变常转移至同侧颈内静脉旁淋巴结群。全身转移少见，除非原发病变已极度进展。
d. 一般而言，早期病变适合放疗，而进展期病变则须手术切除。但有全身转移者则不宜手术。

a. A laryngectomy specimen that has been opened anteriorly. It demonstrates a large mucosal ulcer, which is a squamous cell carcinoma.
b. The vast majority of laryngeal cancers occur in patients who have a history of smoking, commonly associated with significant alcohol intake.
c. Early-stage disease usually remains confined to the larynx. More advanced tumours may metastasize to the ipsilateral anterior triangle jugular chain lymph nodes. Systemic metastases are rare unless the loco-regional disease is very advanced.
d. In general terms, early-stage disease is treated with radiotherapy while advanced disease is treated by surgery.

52. a. 几乎可以肯定病变为鳞状细胞癌。
b. 若不予治疗，病变可发展并累及整个耳廓，甚至侵犯邻近的颞骨。也可能转移至腮腺或乳突淋巴结。
c. 可选择手术或放疗。放疗对外观破坏较小，但可能引起经久不愈的溃疡，特别是在耳廓软骨已暴露的情况下。
d. 最可能的病因是过度日晒。

a. This is almost certainly a squamous cell carcinoma.
b. The lesion will enlarge and infiltrate the rest of the pinna and then the adjacent temporal bone. Metastasis to the parotid or mastoid lymph nodes may also occur.
c. Radiotherapy or surgery is the treatment of choice. Radiotherapy results in less cosmetic disfigurement but may result in a non-healing ulcer, particularly if the tumour has caused cartilage exposure.
d. Prolonged exposure to sunlight.

53. a. 上颌骨全切术。
b. 长期溢泪是由于鼻泪管阻塞导致泪液持续自眼部溢出。
c. 晚期鼻窦癌常可累及邻近结构而出现相关症状。因此晚期上颌窦癌可表现出同侧“胶耳”（鼓室内胶冻状黏稠分泌物）、鼻出血或上列牙齿松动。

a. A radical maxillectomy.
b. This term describes excessive watering of the eye caused by obstruction of the naso-lacrimal duct.
c. Sinus carcinomas usually present late on with symptoms related to involvement of adjacent structures. With regard to maxillary sinus

tumours presentation can take the form of ipsilateral glue ear, epistaxis or development of a loose tooth.

54. a. 声带任克水肿。
   b. 常见病因为甲状腺功能低下、吸烟和过度用声。
   c. 首先应排除甲状腺功能低下。当水肿明显时，应撕除病变黏膜，术后进行嗓音恢复训练。同时应嘱患者戒烟。

   a. Reinke's oedema.
   b. Hypothyroidism, smoking or voice abuse.
   c. Hypothyroidism needs to be excluded. When the oedema is marked the excess mucosa should be trimmed from the vocal cords and the patient referred for speech therapy. Advice must be given regarding cessation of smoking.

55. a. 黑毛舌系由于不明原因的舌乳头良性增生，使舌乳头的外观呈毛发样。
   b. 不严重。尽管毛舌的外观常使患者感到不安，但其并不造成严重后果，亦不会引发其他病变。
   c. 本病无需特殊治疗，但可以用牙刷轻刷舌面以缓解。无需使用抗生素。

   a. Black hairy tongue is due to the colonization of the tongue mucosa by certain non-pathogenic bacteria.
   b. No. Although it causes a great deal of patient concern it is not serious and does not lead on to any other problems.
   c. The condition does not need to be treated but gentle brushing of the tongue, e.g. with a toothbrush, can help. Antibiotics are not indicated.
   d. Tongue cancers usually present with a local ulcer, which may be sore or painful. In a minority cervical lymph node metastases may be the presenting symptom.

56. a. 这是一张牙曲面断层片。
   b. 该片可显示整个下颌及下列牙，并可进行双侧对比。与侧位X平片比较，此种投照避免了双侧下颌骨支的重叠。
   c. 右侧下颌骨体骨质破坏。由于病变边界不规则，故恶性可能性极大。
   d. 本病例不适宜放疗。因为放射线很难消除侵入骨质深层的肿瘤细胞。

a. An orthopantomogram (OPG).
b. It demonstrates the whole mandible and lower jaw dentition and allows comparison of the two sides. It avoids the superimposing of one ramus over the other as can occur with lateral X-rays.
c. Erosion of the horizontal ramus on the right side. This is almost certainly malignant in origin, because of its irregular outline.
d. Radiotherapy would be inappropriate in such a situation as it would be very unlikely to eradicate disease infiltrating the bone.

57. a. 该患者几乎可以确诊为甲状腺肿。
b. 由于甲状腺呈弥漫性肿大，故一般为良性病变。
c. 需行甲状腺 B 超及甲状腺功能检查。
d. 患者可有甲状腺功能亢进或低下等全身表现，亦可有声嘶、吞咽困难。

a. This patient almost certainly has a goitre.
b. Given the generalized enlargement of the gland it is likely to be benign in origin.
c. Ultrasound scan of the thyroid and thyroid function tests.
d. Symptoms of hypo- or hyperthyroidism, hoarseness or dysphagia.

58. a. Sturge-Weber 综合征（脑面血管瘤病）。
b. 由毛细血管异常增生形成的海绵状血管瘤除了沿三叉神经某一分支支配区域分布外，还常累及颅内软脑膜。
c. 患者常有癫痫发作。大多数患者虽然常合并精神障碍和 / 或轻度偏瘫，但往往有多年的生存期。

a. Sturge-Weber syndrome (encephalofacial angiomatosis).
b. As well as a capillary or cavernous haemangioma occupying the distribution of one of the branches of the trigeminal nerve, there is a leptomeningeal angioma intracranially.
c. Epilepsy is common. The majority of patients survive many years, though often with mental defects and/or a hemiparesis.

59. a. 下颌下腺造影检查。
b. 下颌下腺疼痛和 / 或肿胀，常常于进食或饮水时发生。
c. 造影检查常可显示下颌下腺导管慢性阻塞，常由导管狭窄或结石所致。
d. 与下颌下腺密切相邻的神经有：面神经下颌缘支、舌神经及舌下神经。

a. Submandibular gland sialogram.
b. Pain and/or swelling of the submandibular gland, often in association with eating or drinking.
c. Chronic obstruction of the main gland duct, which is usually due to a stenosis or a stone.
d. The marginal mandibular branch of the facial nerve, the lingual nerve and the hypoglossal nerve.

60. a. 充血性心力衰竭。
b. 充血肿大的心脏压迫左侧喉返神经，从而引起左侧声带麻痹，导致声嘶。
c. 比声嘶更为严重的并发症是由于误吸食物或唾液引起的吸入性肺炎。因此问诊时应详细追问吞咽情况。
d. 控制心衰后，可行甲状软骨成形术或患侧声带内聚四氟乙烯树脂（teflon）注射术，以缓解声嘶。

a. Congestive cardiac failure.
b. Such cardiomegaly can cause pressure damage to the left recurrent laryngeal nerve and therefore a vocal cord palsy.
c. More important than the hoarse voice is the risk of aspiration of food or saliva with consequent aspiration pneumonia. The patient should therefore be asked about problems relating to swallowing.
d. Along with the management of the heart failure, consideration should be given to improving laryngeal competence, e.g. by a thyroplasty or Teflon injection of the ipsilateral vocal cord.

61. a. 这是一个气管造瘘口。
b. 造瘘口上方的皮肤缺损，绝大多数与咽腔相通，形成咽瘘。
c. 该并发症易见于营养不良及曾经接受颈部放疗的患者。

a. This is the tracheostome.
b. The upper skin defect almost certainly communicates with the pharynx, forming a pharyngocutaneous fistula.
c. Those with previous nutritional impairment and those who have previously undergone radiotherapy to the neck tissues.

62. a. 靠触诊即可判断肿物为囊性或实性。
b. 核磁共振扫描可以显示肿物与周围软组织的关系。
c. 任何口底的肿物，一旦增大均有导致气道梗阻的风险，因为肿物增大可向后上方压迫并推挤口咽部。

a. By manual palpation.
b. An MRI scan would delineate the mass and its relation to other soft tissue structures in the neck.
c. Any floor of mouth swelling that has the potential to increase in size is a threat to the airway as postero-superior displacement of the oropharynx can cause obstruction.

63. a. 该患者患有典型的声带肉芽肿。此种病变尤其好发于声门后部，常由于杓区黏膜压迫性坏死形成。
b. 当气管内插管的患者在插管后48小时仍不能拔管时，应改行气管造口术，以防止声带肉芽肿形成。
c. 病变可用激光汽化疗法，但极有可能复发。

a. This patient has typical vocal cord granulomas. These characteristically occur in the posterior part of the glottis and result from pressure necrosis of the mucosa overlying the arytenoid cartilages.
b. If a patient is likely to require intubation for longer than 48h, consideration should be given to the creation of a formal or mini tracheostomy.
c. The granulomas can be dealt with by laser vaporization but recurrence can ensue.

64. a. 这是典型的声带小节，常见于职业用声的人群，如歌手。
b. 早期病变通过适当的嗓音训练可望消退。如图中所示般大小的病变，则最好在显微喉镜下切除。
c. 注意用嗓卫生。

a. This is the characteristic appearance of singer's nodules.
b. Early nodules can be reversed by appropriate speech therapy. Nodules as large as those demonstrated are best removed by microlaryngoscopy.
c. Improved speech hygiene.

65. a. 悬雍垂裂。
b. 常合并有硬腭后部的黏膜下缺损及轻度硬腭功能不全。
c. 小儿患者应避免行腺样体切除手术。

a. A bifid uvula.
b. A submucosal cleft in the posterior portion of the bony hard palate with a mild palatal dysfunction.
c. Adenoidectomy in young children should be avoided in such instances.

66. a. 临床上称之为“白斑”，但这并非病理学名词。对口腔白斑患者，应排除口腔念珠菌病。
b. 念珠菌感染引起的白斑，可被棉拭子擦除。否则，只有通过切开式活组织检查方能明确病变性质。
c. 活检常见黏膜上皮一定程度的发育异常。本病常无需特殊治疗。但如果病变严重（如为原位癌），则应行黏膜撕脱术或激光切除。

a. Clinically this is leukoplakia, which in itself is not a pathological diagnosis. It is important to distinguish mucosal abnormalities from oral candidiasis.
b. Having excluded candida (the plaques of which can be removed with a swab) the underlying pathology can only be ascertained by incisional biopsy.
c. Biopsy usually demonstrates a degree of dysplasia of the mucosa. This may not require active treatment but if it is very severe (e.g. carcinoma in situ) then stripping or laser excision of the involved mucosa is required.

67. a. 口腔 - 上颌窦瘘。
b. 牙曲面正位片不仅能显示牙齿的病变，还能明确合并的上颌窦感染。
c. 局部旋转黏膜瓣常可满意修复瘘管。但应在修复前治疗合并的上颌窦感染以确保修复成功。

a. An oro-antral fistula.
b. An OPG X-ray will not only demonstrate the status of the teeth but will also identify any associated infection in the maxillary antrum.
c. The fistula can usually be closed using a local mucosal rotation flap. However, if there is evidence of an associated sinus infection then this will also need to be treated for a successful result.

68. a. 该患者患有颈椎骨髓炎。
b. 此种影像学表现也见于颈椎压缩性骨折及颈椎结核。
c. 需要切除病变椎骨，通过植骨术来稳定颈段脊柱。

a. This patient has osteomyelitis of the cervical spine.
b. A crush fracture or tuberculosis are also possible causes.
c. The spine needs to be stabilized by appropriate bone grafting.

69. a. 肢端肥大症。

b. 糖耐量试验，若实验开始后 2 小时内血生长激素不能降至 2mU/L，则为阳性。除此之外，还应行脑垂体核磁共振扫描，常用钆作对比剂。

c. 首选手术切除，常在鼻内镜下经蝶窦切除。若无法手术，还可用生长抑素类药物保守治疗，或采用放疗。

a. Acromegaly.

b. By a glucose tolerance test, and failure to suppress growth hormone to less than 2mU/l. A pituitary MRI scan should also be performed, preferably with gadolinium contrast enhancement.

c. The treatment of choice is surgery. The gland can be approached trans-sphenoidally. If this is not appropriate then the choice is between treatment with a somatostatin analogue and/or radiotherapy.

70. a. “螺丝钻”样或“胡桃夹”样食管。

b. 该病变由食管神经肌肉功能紊乱导致。患者有吞咽困难，尤其是进流食时；进固体食物时反而较轻。

c. 可有心绞痛样胸痛。

d. 确诊前应当首先排除心脏疾病。应用钙离子阻滞剂（如硝苯地平）后症状缓解，提示为心绞痛可能性大。极少数病例在行食管下段肌肉切开术后可缓解病情。

a. Corkscrew or nutcracker oesophagus.

b. This is a disorder of neuromuscular control of the oesophagus and the patient will have more difficulty swallowing fluids than solids.

c. With angina-like chest pain.

d. It is important to reassure the patient regarding their cardiac status. A calcium entry blocker (e.g. nifedipine) is often helpful. In rare cases a lower oesophageal myotomy can be beneficial.

71. a. 气管造口术。

b. 其适应证为：严重的上气道梗阻、喉功能不全及气管插管后长期不能拔管等。

c. 在小儿，术中可能将颈动脉误认为气管。为防止误切颈动脉，可于造口前用细针穿刺并吸取管内容物以准确判断。小儿气管内径小，因此行气管造瘘时不宜行气管开窗术，而代之以纵行短切口，用缝线固定。

a. Tracheostomy.
b. Upper airways obstruction, protection of the airway for laryngeal incompetence, prolonged intubation.
c. In very young children the carotid artery can be mistaken for the trachea. Aspiration of the contents through a fine-bore needle is a wise precaution before creating a window in the trachea. In children the trachea is of small diameter and a vertical slit with stay sutures, rather than an excised window, should be created for the stoma.

相关词汇英中对照

A

Abiotrophies	功能缺陷
Abscess	脓肿
intracranial	颅内的
parapharyngeal	咽旁的
parotid	腮腺
peritonsillar	扁桃体周的
postauricular	耳后的
retropharyngeal	咽后的
septal	鼻中隔的
subdural	硬膜下的
Accessory auricles	副耳
Accessory nerve palsy	副神经麻痹
Acoustic neuroma	听神经瘤
Acromegaly	肢端肥大症
Acute epiglottitis	急性会厌炎
Acute laryngotracheobronchitis (croup)	急性喉气管支气管炎
Acute mastoiditis	急性乳突炎
Acute otitis media	急性中耳炎
Acute parotid abscess	急性腮腺脓肿
Acute sinusitis	急性窦炎
Adenoids	腺样体
Adrenaline	肾上腺素
Allergic rhinitis	变应性鼻炎
Allergy	变态反应
Angiofibroma	血管纤维瘤
Antihistamines	抗组胺药物
Antral washout	窦腔冲洗
Antrochoanal polyp	上颌窦 - 后鼻孔息肉
Aplasias	发育不全
Artificial larynx	人工喉
Aspergillus spp.	曲霉菌
Aspiration pneumonia	吸入性肺炎

Atrophic rhinitis	萎缩性鼻炎
Audiometry	听力检测法
Auricular prostheses	耳廓假体

B

Basal cell carcinoma	基底细胞癌
Bell's (idiopathic) palsy	(特发性）面瘫
Benign paroxysmal positional vertigo	良性阵发性位置性眩晕
Betamethasone	倍他米松
Bismuth, iodoform and paraffin paste	铋、碘仿和石蜡软膏
Black hairy tongue	黑毛舌
Blood dyscrasias	恶性血液病
Blowout fracture	击出性骨折
Bone anchored hearing aids	骨锚式助听器
Branchial cyst/fistula	腮裂囊肿 / 瘘管
Bronchus, foreign body	支气管，异物
Bullous myringitis	大疱性鼓膜炎

C

Cahart's notches	Cahart 切迹
Caldwell-Luc approach	柯 - 陆氏手术
Caloric testing	冷热水试验
Carcinoma	癌
basal cell	基底细胞
nasopharyngeal	鼻咽
sinus	窦
tongue	舌
see also Squamous cell carcinoma; Tumours	*亦见* 鳞状细胞癌
Catarrh	卡他
Cauliflower ear	菜花耳
Cellulitis	蜂窝织炎
orbital	眶
pinna	耳廓
Cervical lymphadenopathy	颈淋巴结肿大
Children	儿童

laryngeal obstruction	喉阻塞
nasal airway obstruction	鼻气道阻塞
Choanal atresia	鼻后孔闭锁
Cholesteatoma	胆脂瘤
Chordoma	脊索瘤
Chronic otitis media	慢性中耳炎
Chronic sinusitis	慢性鼻窦炎
Cleft lip	唇裂
Cleft palate	腭裂
Cochlear echoes	耳声发射
Cochlear implants	人工耳蜗
Congenital branchial fistula	先天性鳃裂瘘管
Congenital ear disease	耳的先天性疾病
Congenital laryngeal obstruction	先天性喉阻塞
Congenital neck masses	先天性颈部包块
Congestive cardiac failure	充血性心力衰竭
Corkscrew oesophagus	螺丝钻样食管
Cranial nerve palsies	脑神经麻痹
Croup	哮吼
Cyst	囊肿
branchia	鳃裂
pinna	耳廓
thyroglossal	甲状舌管
Cystic hygroma	水囊状淋巴管瘤

D

Dacryocystorhinostomy	鼻泪囊吻合术
Deafness	耳聋
noise-induced	噪声性
rehabilitation	康复
sensorineural hearing loss	感音神经性聋
see also Hearing aids	*亦见* 助听器
Deviated septum	鼻中隔偏曲
Diphtheria	白喉
Diplopia	复视
Double vision	复视
Dressings	填塞物

E

Ear	耳
assessment	检查
congenital disease	先天性疾病
external trauma	外耳创伤
Ear piercing	耳孔
Ear wax	耵聍
Endoscopic surgery	内镜手术
Enephalofacial angiomatosis	脑面部血管瘤病
Epilepsy	癫痫
Epiphora	溢泪
Epistaxis	鼻出血
Epley particle-repositioning manoeuvre	Epley 耳石复位法
Epstein-Barr virus	EB 病毒
Ethmoid sinus	筛窦
Ethmoiditis	筛窦炎
Eustachian tube function	咽鼓管功能
Evoked otoacoustic emissions	耳声发射
Exostoses	外生性骨疣
External auditory canal	外耳道
congenital atresia	先天性闭锁
exostoses	外生性骨疣
stenosis	狭窄
External ear	外耳
furunculosis	疖
trauma	创伤
tumours	肿瘤

F

Facial fractures	面部骨折
Facial nerve monitoring	面神经监测
Facial nerve palsy	面神经麻痹
Facial palsy	面瘫
False fundus	假性外耳道底
Fibre-optic endoscopy	纤维内镜检查
Fistula	瘘管
branchial	鳃裂

oro-antral	口腔 - 上颌窦
pharyncocutaneous	咽瘘
postauricular	耳后
Foreign body	异物
ear	耳
nose	鼻
upper aerodigestive tract	上呼吸消化道
Frontal sinusitis	额窦炎
Functional endoscopic sinus surgery	功能性鼻窦内镜手术
Furunculosis	疖

G

Gentamicin	庆大霉素
Geographic tongue	地图舌
Glossopharyngeal nerve palsy	舌咽神经麻痹
Glucose tolerance test	糖耐量试验
Glue ear	胶耳
Goitre	甲状腺肿
Gradenigo's syndrome	岩尖综合征
Granular myringitis	肉芽性鼓膜炎
Grommets	鼓膜通气管
extrusion of	排出
Gut-associated lymphoid tissue (GALT)	咽淋巴环

H

Haemophilus influenzae	流感嗜血杆菌
Hairy leukoplakia	毛状白斑
Hearing aids	助听器
air conduction	气导
bone anchored	骨锚式
Hereditary haemorrhagic telangiectasia	遗传性出血性毛细血管扩张症
Herpes zoster	带状疱疹
HIV	人类免疫缺陷病毒
Hoarseness	声嘶
Human immunodeficiency virus	人类免疫缺陷病毒
Human papilloma virus	人类乳头瘤病毒
Hyperthyroidism	甲状腺功能亢进

Hypoglossal nerve palsy	舌下神经麻痹
Hypopharynx, foreign body	下咽，异物
Hypothyroidism	甲状腺功能低下

I

Infectious mononucleosis	传染性单核细胞增多症
Inferior turbinate	下鼻甲
Inner ear	内耳
Intracranial abscess	颅内脓肿

K

Kaposi's sarcoma	肉瘤
Kiesselbach's plexus	柯氏静脉丛

L

Labyrinthitis, suppurative	迷路炎，化脓性
Lacrimal sac	泪囊
Laryngeal obstruction	喉阻塞
Laryngeal polyps	喉息肉
Laryngeal tumours	喉肿瘤
Laryngitis	喉炎
Laryngocele	喉膨出
Laryngoscopy	喉镜检查术
Larynx	喉
artificial	人工的
clinical examination	临床检查
diverticula	憩室
Reinke's oedema	任克水肿
Lateral sinus thrombosis	乙状窦血栓形成
Leukoplakia	白斑
Lingual thyroid	舌甲状腺
Little's area	黎氏区
Ludwig's angina	咽峡炎
Lupus pernio	冻疮样狼疮
Lupus vulgaris	寻常狼疮
Lymphoma	淋巴瘤

M

Malleus	锤骨
Mastoidectomy	乳突根治术
Mastoiditis, acute	乳突炎，急性
Maxillary (Le Fort) fractures	上颌骨(Le Fort)骨折
Maxillary sinusitis	上颌窦炎
Maxillectomy	上颌骨切除术
Ménière's disease	梅尼埃病
Meningitis	脑膜炎
Merocel Oto-Wick dressing	外耳道填塞物
Microlaryngoscopy	显微喉镜检查术
Microsurgery	显微手术
Microtia	小耳畸形
Middle ear	中耳
effusions	渗出
microsurgery	显微手术
Mouth	口
diseases of floor	口底疾病
swelling of floor	口底肿胀
see also Tongue	*亦见* 舌
Muco-pyocele	黏脓囊肿
Mucocele	黏液囊肿
Mumps	流行性腮腺炎
Mycobacterium tuberculosis	结核分支杆菌
Myringoplasty	鼓膜成形术

N

Nasal airway obstruction	鼻气道阻塞
Nasal fractures	鼻骨骨折
Nasal packing	鼻腔填塞
Nasal papilloma	鼻乳头状瘤
Nasal polyposis	鼻息肉病
Nasal septum	鼻中隔
deviated	偏曲的
septal abscess	中隔脓肿
septal haematoma	中隔血肿
septal perforation	中隔穿孔

Nasolacrimal duct	鼻泪管
Nasopharyngeal carcinoma	鼻咽癌
Nasopharyngeal tumours	鼻咽肿瘤
Neck masses	颈部包块
Neck space infections	颈部间隙感染
Noise-induced deafness	噪声性聋
Non-allergic rhinitis	非变应性鼻炎
Non-infective rhinitis	非感染性鼻炎
Nose	鼻
clinical examination	临床检查
diseases of	疾病
foreign body	异物
tumours	肿瘤
Nose bleed	鼻出血
Nutcracker oesophagus	胡桃夹样食管

O

Oesophagus	食管
corkscrew (nutcracker)	螺丝钻（胡桃夹）样
foreign body	异物
Olfactory filaments	嗅丝
Optic nerve	视神经
Oral candidiasis	口腔念珠菌病
Orbit, blowout fracture	眶，击出性骨折
Orbital cellulitis	眶蜂窝织炎
Oro-antral fistula	口腔 - 上颌窦瘘
Oropharynx, foreign body	口咽，异物
Orthopantomogram	牙曲面断层片
Osler-Weber-Rendu syndrome see Hereditary haemorrhagic telangiectasia	Osler-Weber-Rendu 综合征 *见* 遗传性毛细血管扩张病
Ossiculoplasty	听骨链成形术
Osteogenesis imperfecta	成骨不全
Osteoma	骨瘤
Osteomyelitis	骨髓炎
Otalgia	耳痛
Otitic barotrauma	耳气压伤

Otitis externa	外耳炎
bacterial	细菌性
dressing	填塞物
fungal	真菌性
necrotizing (malignant)	坏死性（恶性）
Otitis media	中耳炎
acute	急性的
chronic	慢性的
suppurative	化脓的
Otogenic vertigo	耳源性眩晕
Otorrhoea	耳漏
Otosclerosis	耳硬化症
Otoscopy	耳镜检查术

P

Palatal cleft	腭裂
Palatal tumours	腭肿瘤
Palate, diseases of	腭，疾病
Paranasal sinus tumours	鼻窦肿瘤
Parapharyngeal abscess	咽旁脓肿
Parotid gland swellings	腮腺膨大
Pars flaccida	松弛部
Pars tensa	紧张部
attic (marginal) perforation	上鼓室（边缘型）穿孔
central perforation	中央型穿孔
Perichondritis	软骨膜炎
Peritonsillar abscess (quinsy)	扁桃体周围脓肿
Pharyncocutaneous fistula	咽瘘
Pharyngeal diverticula	咽部憩室
Pharyngeal pouch	咽囊
Pinna	耳廓
cellulitis	蜂窝织炎
sebaceous cyst	皮脂腺囊肿
squamous cell carcinoma	鳞状细胞癌
tumours	肿瘤
Pneumococcus spp.	肺炎球菌
Pollen allergy	花粉过敏

Positional testing	位置试验
Postauricular abscess	耳后脓肿
Postauricular fistula	耳后瘘管
Postauricular swelling	耳后肿胀
Postnasal discharge	后鼻孔滴漏
Preauricular sinus	耳前窦道
Proteus spp.	变形杆菌
Pseudomonas spp.	假单胞菌

Q

Quadrilateral cartilage	四方软骨
Quinsy	扁桃体周脓肿

R

Ramsay Hunt syndrome	Ramsay-Hunt 综合征
Ranula	舌下囊肿
Reinke's oedema	任克水肿
Rendu-Osler-Weber syndrome	Rendu-Osler-Weber 综合征
Retropharyngeal abscess	咽后脓肿
Rhinophyma	肥大性酒渣鼻
Rinne test	Rinne 试验

S

Schiebe anomaly	Schiebe 畸形
Schwartze sign	Schwartze 征
Sebaceous cyst	皮脂腺囊肿
Sensorineural hearing loss	感音神经性聋
Septal abscess	鼻中隔脓肿
Septal haematoma	鼻中隔血肿
Septal perforation	鼻中隔穿孔
Sialogram	唾液腺造影
Singer's nodules	声带小结
Sinonasal adenocarcinoma	鼻 - 鼻窦腺癌
Sinus carcinoma	鼻窦癌
Sinusitis	鼻窦炎
acute	急性的
chronic	慢性的

frontal	额窦的
maxillary	上颌（窦）的
Skin grafts, head and neck	皮片，头颈部
Sphenoiditis	蝶窦炎
Squamous cell carcinoma	鳞状细胞癌
ear	耳
mouth	口
nose	鼻
Stapedius muscle	镫骨肌
Stapes prosthesis	镫骨假体
Stomal stenosis	造瘘口狭窄
Streptococcus viridans	溶血性链球菌
Sturge-Weber syndrome	Sturge-Weber 综合征
Subdural abscess	硬膜下脓肿
Subglottic stenosis	声门下狭窄
Submandibular gland	下颌下腺
diseases of	疾病
sialogram	腺管 X 线造影术
Subperichondrial haematoma	软骨膜下血肿
Sudden unilateral vestibular failure	突发性单侧前庭功能障碍
Suppurative labyrinthitis	化脓性迷路炎
Suppurative otitis media	化脓性中耳炎
complications	并发症
Swelling	肿胀
floor of mouth	口底
parotid gland	腮腺
postauricular	耳后
tongue	舌
Swimmers' exostoses	（游泳者）外生性软骨疣

T

Temporal bone fracture	颞骨骨折
Temporalis fascia graft	颞肌筋膜移植片
Thyroglossal cyst	甲状舌管囊肿
Tinnitus	耳鸣
Tongue	舌
benign conditions	良性病变

black hairy	黑毛
carcinoma	癌
swelling	肿胀
tumours	肿瘤
Tonsillar tumours	扁桃体肿瘤
Tonsillitis	扁桃体炎
Torus palatinus	腭隆凸
Tracheostome	气管造瘘口
Tracheostomy	气管造口术
Treacher-Collins syndrome	Treacher-Collins 综合征
Tuberculosis	结核
Tumours	肿瘤
ear	耳
external ear	外耳
laryngeal	喉
nasopharyngeal	鼻咽的
nasopharynx	鼻咽
nose	鼻
palatal	腭的
paranasal sinus	鼻窦
parotid gland	腮腺
pinna	耳廓
submandibular gland	下颌下腺
tongue	舌
tonsil	扁桃体
Tuning fork tests	音叉试验
Tympanic membrane	鼓膜
local conditions	局部疾病
perforation	穿孔
retraction	内陷
Tympanosclerosis	鼓室硬化症

U

Uvula, bifid	悬雍垂，分叉

V

Vagus nerve palsy	迷走神经麻痹

van der Hoeve syndrome	van der Hoeve 综合征
Venous sinus thrombosis	静脉窦血栓形成
Vertigo	眩晕
Vocal cord granuloma	声带肉芽肿
Voice rehabilitation	语音康复
Vomer	犁骨

W

Waardenburg syndrome	Waardenburg 综合征
Weber test	Weber 试验
Wegener's granulomatosis	Wegener 肉芽肿病

Z

Zygomatic (malar) fractures	颧弓骨折